Interest Groups
and Health Care Reform
across the United States

Selected Titles in the American Governance and Public Policy Series

Series Editors: Gerard W. Boychuk, Karen Mossberger, and Mark C. Rom

Interest Groups and Health Care Reform across the United States

Virginia Gray,
David Lowery,
and Jennifer K. Benz

Georgetown University Press
Washington, DC

Library of Congress Cataloging-in-Publication Data
Gray, Virginia, 1945–
   Interest groups and health care reform across the United States / Virginia H. Gray, David Lowery, and Jennifer K. Benz.
      p. ; cm.
   Includes bibliographical references and index.
   ISBN 978-1-58901-989-8 (pbk. : alk. paper)
   I. Lowery, David. II. Benz, Jennifer K. III. Title
   [DNLM: 1. Health Care Reform—United States. 2. Federal Government—United States. 3. Health Policy—United States. 4. Politics—United States. 5. Public Opinion—United States. 6. State Government—United States. WA 540 AA1]

362.1′04250973—dc23

2012037462

∞ This book is printed on acid-free paper meeting the requirements of the American National Standard for Permanence in Paper for Printed Library Materials.

15 14 13   9 8 7 6 5 4 3 2 First printing

Printed in the United States of America

CONTENTS

TABLES AND FIGURES

Figures

PREFACE AND ACKNOWLEDGMENTS

This research was launched by an Investigator Award in Health Policy Research from the Robert Wood Johnson Foundation to Virginia Gray and David Lowery (ID# 047727) in 2003. We were intrigued by the repeated attempts of state governments to offer universal coverage to their citizens and by the backlash against managed care that was manifested in many state regulations, yet at the national level policymakers were still chastened by the defeat of President Bill Clinton's Health Security Act in 1994. The focus of scholarly attention was singularly on this defeat, while hardly anyone noticed what had been happening at the state level both before and after the Clinton debacle. However, passage of health policy reforms by states was truly against all odds, in that the organized interests so often blamed for stopping reform in Washington should have had even more leverage at the state level, according to political science theories. Fortunately, the folks at the Robert Wood Johnson Foundation agreed that we had identified an interesting research question and generously awarded us funds to carry out the three-year investigation.

Along the way we have presented nine convention papers and published seven articles from the larger project. We are greatly indebted to several coauthors of these various articles: Jennifer Benz, Mary Deason, Whitt Kilburn, Justin Kirkland, James Monogan, Jennifer Wolak, Jennifer Sykes, and especially Erik Godwin, our most frequent collaborator. All were graduate students in political science at the University of North Carolina, Chapel Hill, at the time the research was conducted. Variations of some of the models in this book appeared in three prior articles, but new explanatory variables have been added to the book's models as well: Virginia Gray, David Lowery, and Erik K. Godwin, "Public Preferences and Organized Interests in Health Policy: State Pharmacy Assistance Programs as Innovations," *Journal of Health Politics, Policy, and Law* 32 (February 2007): 89–129; Virginia Gray, David Lowery, and Erik K. Godwin, "The Political Management of Managed Care: Explaining Variations in State Health Maintenance Organizations Regulations," *Journal of Health Politics, Policy, and Law* 32 (June 2007): 457–95; and Virginia Gray, David Lowery, James Monogan, and Erik Godwin, "Incrementing toward

Nowhere: Universal Health Care Coverage in the States," *Publius: The Journal of Federalism* 40 (January 2010): 82–113. In addition, we have expended a great deal of effort since March 2010 in reworking the book to take account of the Patient Protection and Affordable Care Act (ACA).

Our scholarship is also informed by our personal experiences with the health care system. Virginia Gray was for many years a happy member of a large nonprofit health maintenance organization in Minnesota, eventually serving as chair of its board of directors, and is now enduring the world of fee-for-service medicine in North Carolina. She is also increasingly interested in the financial stability of the Medicare program, which she used to think was for old folks. In 2004 David Lowery moved to the Netherlands, where he experienced nothing but good things from "socialized medicine"; recently he has moved to Pennsylvania and is not sure yet what kind of health care he has. In 2008 we added Jenny Benz to the team; she lives in Massachusetts, the shining laboratory of state health care reform. Needless to say, we had some great arguments about health care as we wrote this book, but it is stronger for our diverse experiences.

This book had a longer than desirable gestation period, but in the end it was slowed down by a good thing—the passage of the ACA in 2010. This landmark accomplishment of President Barack Obama—and Speaker Nancy Pelosi, who jump-started it at a critical time—necessitated more research, but very worthwhile research indeed. The hundred-year-long effort to pass national health care reform had finally succeeded. We can only hope that its implementation will also succeed; it was off to a good start with the US Supreme Court, led by Chief Justice John Roberts, ruling that the individual mandate and the rest of the act is constitutional under the taxing power of Congress. Only the Medicaid portion of the act was reined in a bit.

INTRODUCTION

Interests and Health Policy

This book is about the politics of interest representation. It is also about health care policy and politics in the American states. But it is first and foremost a book about interest representation. Simply put, there is a deep and profound debate among both academics and citizens about the role interest organizations play in the public policy process (Lowery and Gray 2004b). On the one hand, the press routinely recycles stories of undue influence of narrow, selfish special interest groups, highlighting their privileged position in American politics. In academic discussions, this view is sometimes labeled the transactions perspective because it suggests that much of politics is about the purchasing of public policy. These special interests glide through the supermarket of the public policy process, placing their preferred policies in a market basket, and then proceed to the checkout counter to pay in the currency of campaign contributions, promised employment for politicians in postelectoral careers, or simply favors among overly convivial good old boys (Schattschneider 1960). From this perspective, organized interests pose a direct and material threat to democratic government.

Although this view will certainly be familiar to anyone who pays even cursory attention to politics and public policy, it operates alongside an older, more benign view of interest organizations that is often labeled the pluralist perspective. In this view, organized interests play a vital role in democracy, providing both needed technical information about the consequences of proposed policies and vital political information about their salience to selective publics that are not provided by the electoral process per se (Truman 1951). And even most members of the general public, though normally hypercritical of special interests, have their own heroes among organized interests, whether it be a religious organization opposing abortion, an environmental group fighting global warming, or a professional association defending one's career interests. From this perspective, organized interests are an essential element of democratic politics, focusing and weighing public policies so that politicians can better represent citizens.

One might think that, given two such divergent understandings of how organized interests influence the public policy process, it would be easy to distinguish which one was more valid. But the complexities of this process, and how we are able to study it, are such that two sets of scholars can all too often look at the same basic facts and draw conclusions that are seemingly polar opposites. For example, we know as a factual matter that business interests dominate, at least in terms of simple numbers, the interest communities at both the national and state levels in the United States (Lowery and Brasher 2004). To Kay Schlozman and John Tierney, in *Organized Interests and American Democracy* (1986), the hordes of business lobbyists can only indicate their untoward influence in the public policy process. Recently Schlozman and colleagues reported that this disturbing trend had continued over the past twenty-five years; to paraphrase Schattschneider (1960), the heavenly chorus still sings with an upper-class accent, but the chorus has become larger (Schlozman, Verba, and Brady 2012, 369). To John Heinz, Edward Laumann, Robert Nelson, and Robert Salisbury in *The Hollow Core* (1993), the very presence of such business organizations suggests instead that they are so profoundly disadvantaged by the policy process that they must seek redress via lobbying. Thus, though both the transactions' deeply negative view of the influence of organized interests and the much more positive view of the pluralists are easily distinguished at a theoretical level, bringing data to bear to resolve their debate has proven far from easy.

And there is, of course, a third perspective, sometimes labeled the neopluralist model (Lowery and Gray 2004a), that offers a more complex assessment of the role of organized interests in American politics. To neopluralists, organized interests are sometimes influential in the policy process and sometimes not. It also suggests that there are no permanent arrays of allies and enemies among organized interests. And it suggests that victories or losses are never permanent—winners in the policy process today may become losers tomorrow. This more contingent assessment of the role of organized interests suggests that the *specific* nature of the issue matters a great deal. Is a *specific* issue salient and popular among citizens? In what venue is the *specific* issue being decided? How does the *specific* issue mobilize *specific* combinations of supporters and opponents among organized interests? And how are these combinations arrayed against each other over these *specific* issues in different political contexts? Thus, this perspective suggests that we need to go beyond looking at who is present within lobbying communities to look at how specific configurations of organized interests engage each other over quite precise policy proposals in different political contexts.

And that is why this book is also a health care policy book and a book on American state politics. With regard to the first, health care policy offers us a complex set of policy choices over an array of specific issues. We will see that efforts to reform the health care system have been remarkably successful at some times and in some places, most notably in some of the American states, and have been a complete failure at other times and places. In some places and on some occasions, public support for health care reform has been quite strong; and in other settings, it has been remarkably less so. We will also see that some health care issues generate patterns of allies and enemies that are markedly different than others, with allies on some issues becoming enemies on others. This pattern of variation provides us an enticing arena in which to assess the relative importance of hypothesized determinants of the success or failure of proposed policy reforms. And among those hypothesized determinants, of course, are organized interests. And here, too, examining health care policy offers a nearly ideal focus for our analysis of the influence of organized interests. Indeed, we will see that during the last two decades stretching from the failed efforts of President Bill Clinton to adopt a program of national health insurance to President Barack Obama's more successful effort, organized interests have been a central part of the story of public policy on health care—widely credited, for example, with effectively stopping reform at the national level in the 1990s. In short, the story of health care policy in the United States over the last two decades offers us an important lens through which to assess when and how organized interests might influence public policy.

Still, if we restrict our attention to the divergent Clinton and Obama records on universal health care, we would still lack the empirical bite needed to rigorously assess the contingent expectations of the neopluralist view of organized interests. Universal health care, after all, is only one type of health care policy, albeit a very significant and encompassing one. Moreover, the Clinton and Obama experiences offer us only two observations on the kinds of contextual forces that neopluralists suggest might matter in determining whether organized interests are successful or not in influencing public policy. And this is why this is also a book on state politics. During the years before and between the two national-level cases, the states explored a wide range of health care proposals, with many different kinds of reforms being adopted in many states. Thus, in the states we have a variation of policies unmatched at the national level. And this variation in policy proposals is matched by variations in the institutional and political contexts of the states, differences in context that we must account for if we are to assess the unique influence of organized interests in the public policy process. And just as important, scholars have long studied the policy process of the American states, a history that provides us with powerful theories and techniques, most notably diffusion analysis, with which to untangle the role of organized interests in health care policy.

So, again, this is foremost a book on organized interests, but it is also a book on health care policy and American state politics. We begin in chapter 1 to meld these three topics by first examining the history of health care reform in the United States at both the national and state levels. We then examine the kinds of data at the state level on health policy and organized interests that we use to assess the complex and contingent role of organized interests in health care policymaking. And finally, we introduce the range of theories and methods used to assess the role of competing influences on public policymaking in the American states.

CHAPTER 1

Health Care and Organized Interests in the United States

Universal health care coverage was on the national political agenda for nearly a hundred years, from the platform of Teddy Roosevelt's Bull Moose Party in 1912, to President Franklin Roosevelt's consideration in the 1930s, to the long string of presidents who introduced major reform bills to expand access—starting with Harry Truman in the 1940s, to Lyndon Johnson, who got Medicare and Medicaid adopted in 1965; continuing with Richard Nixon, who introduced a universal coverage plan subsequently endorsed by Gerald Ford; and to Bill Clinton, whose universal coverage plan based on managed competition failed in 1994. None of their proposals ever reached consideration on the floor of the US Congress. Not until a comprehensive health reform bill supported by President Barack Obama reached the floor of the US House of Representatives on Christmas Eve 2009 did a universal coverage bill (or near-universal, in this case) get so far in the congressional process. Thus the passage of the Patient Protection and Affordable Care Act (ACA) in March 2010 was truly a landmark accomplishment. In the punctuated equilibrium framework offered by Baumgartner and Jones (1993), we observed nearly a hundred years of stability within the health policy subsystem, interrupted only by the addition of Medicaid and Medicare in the 1960s, and then finally in 2010 we had a dramatic punctuation in this equilibrium. To be sure, the federal government had made a couple of incremental adjustments that increased coverage for specific groups, namely, the Children's Health Insurance Program (CHIP), which was enacted in 1997 for children, and Medicaid's 1115 waiver program, which affects clients who meet state and federal eligibility criteria.[1] But neither program purports to be a *universal* coverage program for *all* citizens.

At the point of this writing in December 2012, we do not know how the ACA will play out, given that the Republicans opposed its passage and are placing obstacles in front of its implementation. The new law passed a critical first hurdle when the individual mandate and its associated features, such as state exchanges and consumer protections/insurance regulations, were declared constitutional by the US Supreme Court in June 2012.[2] However, the Medicaid expansion was changed from mandatory to a state choice, albeit a sweet one in which states receive a 100 percent match through 2019 and then 90 percent thereafter. One sign of an implementation problem was that the attorneys general of twenty-six states, all of them Republican, filed or joined lawsuits that wound up at the US Supreme Court, seeking to dismantle the individual mandate, the insurance exchanges, and the extension of Medicaid. Now these same states are being relied upon to implement the state exchanges, which most had not started planning by the late fall of 2012, and to implement the addition of many new patients onto the Medicaid rolls, to which many of them are opposed. Given the Republicans' unified control of twenty-four state governments after the 2012 elections, they should be able to continue to pursue a policy of noncooperation at the state level, such as not participating in the exchanges and entering into Interstate Healthcare Freedom Compacts. However, the ACA's future was secured when Barack Obama was reelected president in November 2012 and the Democrats retained control of the US Senate. At that point the ACA became the law of the land in a way that it had not been in 2010. Hopefully, it will be a true punctuation that reforms the health care system.

The States' Record on Health Care Reform

If instead of a singular focus on what was happening or not happening in Washington during the last century, what if we look one level down—to what the states were doing in health policy? How stable were the health policy subsystems in the fifty states in contrast to the national system? Universal coverage was first adopted by the state of Hawaii in 1974; in the few years before and after the failure of the Clinton plan, the states were very active players in universal coverage: Seventeen states enacted some step toward universal coverage by 2002. In the first decade of this century Maine (2003), Vermont (2006, 2011), and Massachusetts (2006) enacted new universal coverage laws, while at the national level the "public option" proposed in 2010 did not fare so well. It lies buried in the congressional graveyard, leaving some 23 million people without health care access under the 2010 law (Oberlander 2010, 1116). And in 2011 Vermont made history by creating the nation's first "single-payer" health system, Green Mountain Care, to be implemented in 2013 once funding is identified. Thus, the states' record on providing and attempting to provide universal care during the past forty years merits scholarly attention, as least as much as the national government's failure until 2010 has captivated scholars' imagination.

During the same forty-year period the rise and fall of managed care has been one of the most important health care developments in the United States. By the 1990s a backlash against stricter forms of managed care had set in across the country. Congress repeatedly failed to produce any *broad* patient protection legislation, aside from the 1996 Health Insurance Portability and Accountability Act (HIPAA), while all fifty states were active in the regulation of managed care and in offering other ways to protect patients. These state laws, enacted in a backlash against managed care organizations, included new rights for consumers, such as the right to sue, and new limitations on providers and health plans. Legislation in this area diffused quickly across the states in the middle to late 1990s, in what appeared to be a bandwagon effect.

In a third important area of state activity, thirty-four states provided their low-income seniors with financial assistance for their prescription drug bills before the federal government could manage to add that benefit to Medicare, partially in 2003 under President George W. Bush, and fully by 2020 under the ACA. These pharmaceutical programs are of a more routine nature, less conflictual than "whipping HMOs [health maintenance organizations] into shape" and less costly than offering health care to all citizens; yet they are welfare programs, and as such should be expected to generate some opposition. Thus, in contrast to the national level, the state-level health policy subsystem does not appear to be in equilibrium, at least not in the past forty years. Rather, this quick summary of the three health reforms we study in the chapters that follow suggests many punctuations by universal coverage enactments, HMO regulations, and the provision of financial assistance to low-income seniors for prescription drug coverage. Thus studying policymaking activities at the state level, as we do in this book, is likely to be far more illuminating about the role of health interests than studying them at the national level, where basically little but gridlock happened, especially with regard to universal coverage, for one hundred years.

Ours is not necessarily a popular position, given that analysis of nonevents at the national level (e.g., "why no national health insurance?") has consumed the bulk of scholarly attention to health reform, in contrast to relatively sparse research at the state level. Research on state health reform in fact exists only in scholarly journals and in edited books published in the 1990s, with Hackey and Rochefort's 2001 edited volume on reforms in state health policy being the most recent one. To the best of our knowledge, this book is the first scholarly examination of state health reforms from a political science perspective in more than twenty years. Thus, here we are necessarily plowing new ground.

Why National Health Care Reform Now?

It is of course also intriguing to analyze why a policy punctuation in the form of the ACA did occur at the national level in 2010, especially because it will be carried out by the states. Although the scholarly analysis of the enactment of the ACA is far from complete, no doubt much of it will center on the differences between Clinton's failure and Obama's success in achieving major reform.

Before 2010, the canonical story about the lack of health care policy reform was about an undersized David of public interest waging an uphill struggle against the Goliath of big interests. This story is a standard explanation for the failure of Clinton's plan in 1994. Scholars such as Jamieson (1994), West, Heith, and Goodwin (1996), West and Loomis (1999), Weissert and Weissert (2002), and Quadagno (2005), and journalists such as Johnson and Broder (1996), assigned primary blame for the 1994 fiasco to powerful interests representing the health care industry. So scholars with an interest group lens will presumably look toward changes in interest group composition between 1994 and 2010 or to Obama's strategy in dealing with organized interests as possible reasons for the passage of reform in 2010. Even scholars identifying other culprits—the president's strategy somehow "boomeranged" (Skocpol 1996) or "It's the institutions, stupid!" (Steinmo and Watts 1995), policy feedback limits the United States to only incremental reforms (Mayes 2004), or ideology and the sheer complexity of the institutions of the American health care industry (Starr 2011)—agreed that one consequence of their preferred culprit's culpability was to yield enormous power to intransigent organized interests.

Still other scholars (e.g., Peterson 1995; Baumgartner and Talbert 1995) focused more specifically on the internal structure of Congress as the reason for the demise of the Clinton plan; they argued that fragmentation of jurisdictional control over health policy in Congress set up a situation whereby special interests could become more entrenched. Interestingly, one set of congressional scholars (Brady and Kessler 2010) predicted during the height of the reform debate (in a piece published in April 2010) that the outcome for Obama would likely be the same as for Clinton—defeat. They used gridlock theory to show that the Clinton proposal was far to the left of the median House member or the pivotal Senate member, thereby dooming it to failure in 1994. They then showed that the basic conditions remained the same in 2010:

Public opinion was about the same as in 1994; the party lineup in each chamber of Congress was almost exactly the same in 2010 as in 1994 and hence the gridlock regions remained the same; but the economy was in much worse shape in 2010 than in 1994 (Brady and Kessler 2010). Such a pessimistic analysis so late in the legislative game just underscores how skillful President Obama and Democratic legislative leaders were in accomplishing this victory.

In early analyses of the ACA's passage, scholars have continued the theme of analyzing organized interests and institutions, but they often credit President Obama with more skillfully managing negotiations among competing interests and in shepherding legislation through institutions with many veto points. Lawrence Jacobs (2010), for example, stresses the importance of the deals that the president and Democratic leaders cut with medical providers, medical manufacturing groups, and pharmaceutical manufacturers in exchange for their vocal support or silence on the bill, a view echoed by Quadagno (2011), Brown (2011), and Hacker (2011). Jacobs and Skocpol (2010) say that some of these stakeholder groups even contributed to advertising campaigns promoting reform; conversely, they argue that Obama never had to suffer all-out unified opposition from the business community.[3] Peterson (2011) rates both the interest group and institutional prospects as more auspicious for President Obama than for any other president since Franklin Roosevelt, but he also lauds Obama's leadership in exploiting the opportunity. Overall, the triumph over or accommodation to health industry interests (Gibson and Singh 2012) as a compelling reason for the ACA's passage seems to be a central theme in the scholarly analysis of the reform's enactment.

Relatively less emphasis is placed on institutional features as a factor in the bill's passage, but institutional constraints, such as the presence of the filibuster in the Senate, shaped the bill's final content, eliminating the public option and substituting state insurance exchanges for a national exchange (Hacker 2010). Other institutional scholars credited the more centralized and partisan legislative process, called "unorthodox lawmaking," that congressional Democrats borrowed from the Republicans, for the Democrats' victory on health care reform (Beaussier 2012). Still others saw the ACA as just the latest example of delegated governance in which there is only a limited increase in federal governing authority, while most responsibility for the administration and delivery of social programs is shifted away from the federal level to private agents or subnational governments (Morgan and Campbell 2011a). Delegation is seen as a way to overcome institutional barriers to reform.

Figure 1.1 Lobbyists by Health Subsector, 1998–2009

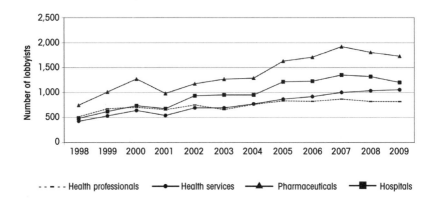

Source: Calculated by the authors from data at opensecrets.org.

Health Care Interests in Washington

From this quick survey of the literatures on both President Clinton's failure and President Obama's success, it is evident that the interest-based approach taken in this book on the states is compatible with one at the national level. It is clear that health interests, once mobilized for the 1994 battle, stayed in Washington, resulting in partisan gridlock over patient protection legislation and Medicare prescription drug benefits for the next decade. Figure 1.1 shows this trend. The number of health industry lobbyists registered to lobby on all health issues totaled 790 in 1998, with all four health industries relatively equal in numbers. There was an inflection point in 2004, when the number of groups increased until 2007 for hospitals and pharmacies. Health services, conversely, increased in a steadily linear fashion through 2009, whereas health professions were more stable across the twelve-year period.[4] Reported lobbying expenditures by health industry groups for the 1998–2010 period totaled nearly $4 billion (Center for Responsive Politics data reported by Hacker 2010, 865).

Lobbying on the ACA was the most intense phase of this period. As seen in figure 1.2, which displays all types of organizations lobbying, not just health groups, 1,880 organizations were registered to lobby on health care reform by the final weeks of the debate in Washington—a nearly fivefold increase from the previous year. Many groups outside health care lobbied, especially business groups such as the US Chamber of Commerce, the National Association of Realtors, and individual corporations, as well as welfare and human rights

Figure 1.2 Federal Lobby Registrations for Health Reform, 2009–10

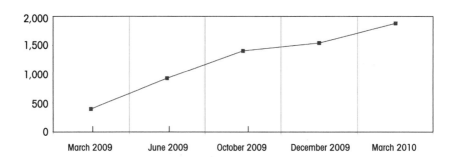

Note: These data come from the Center for Responsive Politics. Rather than listing the groups that lobby on a specific bill, CRP has also listed groups registered to lobby by keyword, such as "healthcare reform," or by bill number and bill title. The key words used to create the search for the first quarter of 2010 were: HR 3200, S. 1796, HR 3962, HR 3590, "affordable health," "healthy future," "health care for America," "health insurance reform," "healthcare reform," "health care reform," and "patient protection" and "Affordable care." They were obtained from Michael Beckel, author of the article found at www.opensecrets.org/news/2010/03/number-of-special-interest-groups-v.html. The other four quarters were obtained from this article.

Source: Calculated by the authors.

advocacy groups, and tribal nations. In 2009 the health care industry spent more than $500 million on lobbying, while the Chamber of Commerce spent $144 million (Hacker 2010, 865, 873).

The Research Puzzle of This Book

The adoption of health policy reform legislation at the state level has been relatively successful compared with the national level, where comprehensive reform had often failed until adoption of the ACA in March 2010. Policy changes in many states in at least three important areas of health policy—universal coverage, regulation of managed care, and financial assistance to seniors for prescription drugs—kept reformers' hopes alive. Although organized interests have been blamed for blocking reform in Washington for nearly one hundred years, the same interests exist in the fifty state capitals, where successful reforms have nonetheless been achieved. This is the central research puzzle of this book.

The fact that state governments took action on health policy in spite of opposing interest forces where the national government did not offers a compelling puzzle that could be studied in a variety of ways. Our approach is to try to understand why the states took action at all and to capitalize on the variation among states in reforms attempted and achieved. The fact that some states took action while others did not offers us variation and affords us the opportunity to test explanations about why some legislatures tackle policy problems and others do not. In particular, we can leverage the institutional variation of the fifty state legislatures and the variation of fifty state interest group systems in our analyses. Further, because states responded with different levels of regulatory stringency and generosity of benefits, we also have the opportunity to test explanations of these dimensions. These are not investigative opportunities that scholars have available at the national level where they are faced with a sample size of one. With the variation provided by the states, we are able to take some of the major explanations for reform failures, such as opposition by organized interests and institutional gridlock, and test them systematically at the state level—something that scholars of national reform are not able to do.

In this chapter we introduce the major state-level health care reforms that we study in this volume—pharmacy assistance, managed care regulation, and universal coverage. Analysis of these three policy areas is the focus of chapters 3, 4, and 5, in which we compare the states' successes with the federal government's lack of success or slowness to succeed. We also outline how the 2010 federal law enacted by Congress and upheld by the Supreme Court will affect the states and how the states' capacities in turn will determine how well or how poorly Obama's plan will be implemented. In this chapter we also discuss the differences between the two governmental levels in the structure of their interest group systems and the relative importance of health care within those systems. The major theoretical perspectives of the book are also discussed. Innovation theory, including internal determinants and external determinants that are critical to explaining the adoption of state health policy innovations, is the focus of this chapter. We outline the concepts from innovation theory that are used in our empirical analyses in chapters 3, 4, and 5. The other major theoretical perspective of the book is population ecology theory, including the density and diversity of organized interests, and this is the focus of chapter 2, in which we list and discuss some of the concepts about interest groups that we employ in our empirical models.

National Reforms versus State Reforms

The story of the power of special interests is even applied to nominally successful efforts to reform the health care system, such as the addition of prescription drug coverage to Medicare in 2003. The fact that Congress debated this bill for nearly a decade, passing a convoluted and inadequate plan only in 2003, is commonly ascribed to the power of lobbyists representing the pharmaceutical industry, health plans, employers, and medical providers, most of which come out way ahead under the Medicare Prescription Drug, Improvement, and Modernization Act of 2003. The Senate minority leader, Democrat Tom Daschle, charged that "this is basically a corporate welfare bill for drug companies and HMOs. We estimate that about one-quarter of all senior citizens will be worse off virtually the day this bill passes" (Serafini 2003). Indeed, health interests were said to be so powerful that they overrode with ease other reputably influential organized interests: Democrats suspicious about the "privatizing" elements in the Medicare bill and antitax conservatives who were upset about an expensive new entitlement. Each of these interests preferred very different kinds of legislation to address the high costs of prescriptions, with liberal Democrats preferring across-the-board coverage for all Medicare recipients, not the introduction of means testing and the confusion over "doughnut holes" in coverage.[5]

In 2010 President Obama secured the support of the Pharmaceutical Research and Manufacturers of America up front with their promise of $80 million during a period of ten years in exchange for a negotiated limit on the burdens to be placed on the pharmaceutical industry. The industry won concessions such as no importation of drugs from Canada and no new rebates on drugs for Medicare patients (Spatz 2010), and it ended up absorbing some of the costs of closing the Part D doughnut hole by 2020.

State Pharmacy Assistance Programs for Needy Seniors

Given the swirl of organized interests in Washington around drug coverage for seniors, it may surprise some that by 2004, thirty-four of the fifty states had already established programs providing prescription drug assistance to low-income seniors. Such programs were targeted at the near-poor elderly (and sometimes the disabled) who did not qualify for Medicaid. Maine and New Jersey were the first to provide drug coverage for their seniors in 1975. Other states enacted drug legislation by the end of the 1980s; the drug assistance movement was then quiescent until 1996. But it took off again, with twenty states adopting prescription drug policies between 1996 and 2004, most before 2001. And adopting these policies was not a one-time event on the states' part. Between 1996 and 2004 many states enacted laws expanding their original pharmacy assistance programs, usually making them more generous. Between 2000 and 2004 three states expanded their programs a second time. Even after passage of Medicare Part D in 2003, leaders of both parties in the states with the most generous policies pledged to maintain them. Referring to the new federal program, a New York Republican senator said, "We are not going to push our senior population into an inferior program" (quoted by Hernandez and Pear 2004, 12). Two weeks before the Medicare drug bill was signed by President Bush, Pennsylvania's governor signed a bill with broad bipartisan support increasing enrollment in the state's program by 100,000 citizens. Since the enactment of Part D in 2003, seven states have started their own new programs of pharmacy assistance to seniors, while fewer states have ceased such programs; however, the most common action has been for states to create or convert existing pharmacy assistance programs to Medicare wraparound programs (2010c). Twenty-three states have taken this action, which provides secondary coverage to low-income seniors for drug expenses not covered by Medicare Part D, such as those incurred in the "doughnut hole."[6]

So why did states, which were already spending heavily on health care programs like Medicaid, decide to offer pharmacy benefits to low-income seniors?[7] It is not as if needy seniors are a mobile group poised to exit for another state, nor is this a benefit designed to attract new residents with skills badly needed in the workforce.[8] In a "race to the bottom" world where the states seemingly compete to offer low taxes and to provide meager welfare benefits, why are they voluntarily financing some of the costs of prescriptions for seniors not quite in poverty? Further, the health of seniors has traditionally been a federal responsibility under Medicare via its link to Social Security. Quite clearly, it was Medicare's original failure to cover prescription drugs in the first place that created the demand for the states to assist elderly citizens. Yet, states continue to help, even as Medicare Part D is enriched. But it is an interesting question as to why thirty-four states have been seemingly so generous with their senior citizens.

However, this simple fact begs the underlying question posed by the traditional explanation of the failure of health care reform at the federal level: Why were the same special interests that were so effective in delaying meaningful prescription drug coverage at the national level, then shaping its final passage so as to disproportionably benefit themselves in 2003, and then delaying the full implementation of the 2010 ACA until 2020, so incapable of stopping the majority of states from passing similar legislation? Why were advocacy groups pushing for prescription coverage unsuccessful for so long in Washington, yet victorious in state capitals? What is different about the number and balance of interest organizations in the states?

To be sure, not all states have adopted prescription drug programs. And among those offering financial help, some reduced their commitment due to budgetary problems in the 2002–4 period or due to the availability of Medicare Part D funds. But when compared with the efforts of the federal government during the last forty years, states' efforts to assist seniors with the costs of prescription drugs are impressive and deserve our scholarly attention. Moreover, the variation in effort among the states allows us to test a number of hypotheses about the determinants of health policy reform, which a sample size of one in Washington does not allow.

Anti–Managed Care Regulations

The story of a gridlocked Washington besieged by intransigent interests unable to deal with a policy problem was repeated again in the case of crafting regulations for managed care. By the late 1960s managed care had become the preferred option of many consumer advocates interested in a greater emphasis on preventive care, and in the next decade it attracted favor with businesses interested in controlling health care costs. This seemingly happy confluence of interests led to such a rapid expansion of managed care that by the 1990s most Americans with private health insurance received care through managed care organizations. But the last decade of the twentieth century was not an easy one for the managed care concept. The incentives for HMOs to control costs came to be seen as antithetical to consumers' interests in the quality of care and in choice of providers. The political response to this changing environment was not long in coming. During the middle to late 1990s, the states—and the federal government, too—considered a variety of proposals to rein in what were perceived as out-of-control HMOs. But only the states were successful in imposing a wide range of regulations on the operation of managed care organizations, including the establishment of new rights for consumers and the application of new limitations on providers.

We take advantage of the variation among states in enacting regulations to discover why some governments are able to address what are often perceived of as intractable policy problems—intractable in a political, not in a true policy, sense. Indeed, we are especially interested in the role that organized interests played in accounting for why some states were aggressive in regulating HMOs while others lagged behind. Why did organized interests stop such legislation in Washington, but not in the fifty states? Not until the ACA of 2010 did the US Congress manage to incorporate meaningful patient protections into federal law, and by then they were aimed at all types of health insurance, not just that for managed care.

Universal Coverage Legislation

Thus far we have two examples of health reforms where state governments managed to triumph over interest group opposition to enact policy reforms. But the state level as a whole was not much more successful than the federal government through 2009 in achieving a third reform—the goal of universal coverage. However, even what looks like a policy failure on the face of it upon closer scrutiny demonstrates that the states' record on universal coverage is still better than the federal level's long policy equilibrium not punctuated until 2010. At the time the Clinton bill was being debated in 1994, seven states had already enacted universal coverage (though most of the seven never implemented it). By 1996 seventeen states had adopted some kind of universal coverage legislation, albeit some for limited or experimental purposes, and legislatures in forty-two states had at least considered it. And as important as President Obama's legislative achievement is in reforming many aspects of health policy and health insurance, the 2010 law will still leave more than 20 million people uninsured and thus is not fully universal. And its implementation depended upon the Democrats' retaining the presidency and/or a majority in the US Senate in November 2012.

We have assembled a unique fifty-state data set that records all instances of universal coverage policy activity by states from 1988 to 2002, the period covered by our interest group data set. Our analysis of the states' steps to expand universal insurance coverage—studies commissioned, bills considered, bills passed by one or both chambers, and bills enacted into law and signed by the governor—allows us to record how far in the legislative process these various measures proceeded. This is truly an original data set that no one else has ever put together.

What kinds of measures count as universal coverage? Although most people probably think of universal coverage as entailing a single-payer plan, like Canada's, when health policy experts used the term "universal health insurance," it applies more generally to *any effort to provide health insurance to all citizens*.[9] Our analyses include only proposals that state a goal of universal coverage and that provide an actual comprehensive plan or at least a legal framework of voluntary and mandatory steps to be enacted, funded, and implemented. Operationally, the Intergovernmental Health Policy Project, now defunct, and the National Conference of State Legislatures (NCSL) judged five types of state legislation as encompassed within universal coverage. One type focused on controlling the costs of health insurance by regulating the market; another mandated employers to cover their employees' insurance. Another type of universal coverage legislation used state funds to set up health insurance programs for needy families and adults without children who do not qualify for Medicaid because they are slightly above the federal poverty line. In some cases, people of modest means can buy into the program by paying a sliding-scale premium. The more far-reaching programs combined all three elements—cost controls, employer mandates, and state funding. The most comprehensive system is a single-payer plan, but none was adopted in the period of our study, though Vermont has done so since then. Still, the states have taken various steps during the last four decades toward universal coverage, even if success remains elusive in the end.

Universal coverage, even if a less successful reform for the states than anti–managed care regulation or pharmacy assistance for seniors, offers several opportunities for our research. First, we want to know if the same interest group forces credited with impeding universal coverage reform at the national level have also limited state efforts to promote universal coverage. Second, we want to understand why these forces are able to impede universal coverage policies at both levels, if they do, but not other health policy reforms that have been enacted at the state level. Third, we seek to develop a systematic explanation of legislative support for universal coverage policies that goes beyond case studies of a handful of adopters. The existing knowledge base rests upon case studies of a handful of states, while laws were actually passed in seventeen states and considered in forty-two states. The unique fifty-state data set we assembled records all instances of universal coverage policy activity in the states beginning in 1988 so that broad-based models can be developed and tested. It allows us to compare interest group effects and institutional effects on advancing or deterring health reform over several years.

Fourth, between the failure of the Clinton Plan in 1994 and the passage of Obama's ACA in 2010, incrementalism again seemed the preferred path for reformers at both the state and national levels. The only expansion of coverage Congress could muster was the Children's Health Insurance Program (CHIP) in 1997, a joint federal–state program for uninsured families with children with incomes just above the Medicaid eligibility line. There is a debate in the policy literature over whether such incremental steps take us anywhere. Does policy activity in the past, even small steps toward a policy goal, make it more likely that full-fledged policy reform will follow (Berkman and Reenock 2004)? Or, as suggested by Baumgartner and Jones (1993, 2002; also see Jones, Sulkin, and Larsen 2003), does real policy reform require a punctuation in which comprehensive universal coverage laws will rapidly diffuse across the states? In this regard, how do we assess the burst of state policy activity beginning in 2003, when Maine adopted its Dirigo Plan and California enacted an employer mandate, only to see it repealed the next year by its voters in a ballot referendum? Then, somewhat unexpectedly, in 2006 Vermont and Massachusetts enacted laws to create universal health coverage for their residents starting in 2007; the Bay State's use of the individual mandate encouraged the federal government to adopt its own mandate in 2010. And in 2011 Vermont decided to enact a single-payer system. However, though reformers continued to introduce universal coverage bills in state legislatures, most states followed the incremental strategy of expanding existing public programs, such as Medicaid via 1115 waivers and CHIP. By 2009 even those efforts were in peril due to the grim budget situation in most states.

At the national level the policy punctuation in health care came with the 2010 passage of the ACA, which broke the long equilibrium dating back to Teddy Roosevelt, President Truman, or to President Johnson's signing of Medicaid and Medicare in 1965, depending on exactly how one counts our history.[10] The 2010 law attempts universal coverage through a variety of means, including expanding Medicaid, requiring individuals and small businesses to buy insurance, providing subsidies for those who cannot afford to do so, and establishing state insurance exchanges where consumers and small businesses can shop. According to estimates by the Congressional Budget Office, by 2019 the number of uninsured American will drop by 32 million; of those left uninsured, about one-third will be illegal immigrants and the rest will be people who do not take advantage of any of the programs mentioned above. The ACA was comprehensive in scope, going well beyond near-universal access to include insurance market regulations (e.g., no annual or lifetime limits on coverage, youth allowed to remain on parents' insurance plan until age twenty-six), differential encouragement to employers to offer insurance (i.e., large businesses will have to pay a tax if they do not offer employees health insurance, whereas small businesses will receive tax credits if they do offer employees insurance), a new long-term care insurance program (since dropped due to design flaws), changes to Medicare (e.g., beginning to close the "doughnut hole" in 2010, and completely closing it in 2020, reducing the financial subsidies to Medicare Advantage plans) and other public programs, and funding for various demonstration and pilot projects. To some, the ACA did not go far enough: It is not a single-payer system; it does not restructure the health care system; rather, the law builds upon the current employer-based system, filling in gaps, and motivating behavior through a mixture of positive and negative incentives. Yet, given the fears of "death panels" and "socialism" shouted out in opposition in 2009, the ACA was surely as much as the American political system would allow in 2010.

Like other major punctuations, this law is likely to set off further policy changes, including for the states. The ACA offers the states considerable flexibility and choices. First, if substantial public sentiment exists in favor of a "public option," then a state could create and offer such a program in its new insurance exchange, according to Halpin and Harbage (2010); it could even be a single-payer system (Jost 2010). So by no means does the federal law stop a state from acting to provide access to coverage for all its citizens in the way it wants. Second, the ACA does not set up a new overarching federal agency to administer the law, but rather offers the states the choice of implementing the law within federal standards or leaving it up to the Department of Health and Human Services to administer the law.[11] Initially, the states were also tasked with establishing high-risk insurance pools by July 1, 2010, for adults with preexisting medical conditions.[12]

More generally, states were given important implementation responsibilities in three major areas: creating new Medicaid eligibility rules that could increase enrollment in the program by as much as 50 percent; modifying a host of existing insurance market regulations to fit with the 2010 law and then providing greater oversight of proposed insurance rate increases; establishing and operating two insurance exchanges, one for small businesses and one for individuals, plus a myriad of other responsibilities (Weil and Scheppach 2010). The US Supreme Court greatly complicated the first decision as it removed the federal coercive power over states that forced them to participate in the expanded Medicaid program for which the federal government will pay at first 100 percent and then later 90 percent of the expenses. Instead, the Supreme Court said that the newly expanded Medicaid program was voluntary for states. Some states' governors are saying that they will refuse to be a part of the expanded part of Medicaid, thus leaving many poor people uncovered in their state. Much of the success of the federal reform depends upon state expertise in health policy administration, the vigor of their insurance enforcement, and whether they embrace the coverage of millions of poor people through expanded Medicaid.

The ACA encountered negative policy feedback from some states, from one even before passage. Virginia became the first state to enact, on March 10, 2010, a new statute titled "Health Insurance Coverage Not Required" (NCSL 2010b). At least twenty-six state attorneys general, nearly all Republicans, joined the Florida lawsuit asking the courts to declare the federal law uncon-stitutional, arguing that the Constitution does not grant Congress the power to require all Americans to carry insurance (Adamy and Perez 2010). In a separate lawsuit, the attorney general of Virginia invoked its nullification stat-ute in an attempt to prevent enforcement (Jost 2010). Although the weight of legal opinion at the time suggested that such challenges had questionable legal merit (Jost 2010; Dorf 2009a, 2009b; for a contra opinion, see Shapiro 2010), they did provide a visible way for the Republican Party to continue to voice its opposition to the new policy. At the least, the legal challenges from states indicate that full implementation of the federal law may vary from state to state, depending upon party control. The US Supreme Court decided the Florida case on June 28, 2012, in *National Federation of Independent Business et al. v. Sebelius*, upholding the constitutionality of the individual mandate as a tax and essentially setting up two Medicaid programs—the present fifty-state program with its varying state matches and a new expanded Medicaid program with enhanced matching that states can opt into if they wish.

An Introduction to Health Interest Communities at the National and State Levels

Our search for an explanation for why health reforms were achieved sooner at the state level than at the national level starts with organized interests, the culprit often blamed at the national level. As noted already, a substantial mo-bilization of health care interests occurred during the battle over President Clinton's Health Security Plan in 1993–94; and those interests, once mobi-lized, stayed in Washington, allegedly making other health reforms difficult to enact. So it might be reasonable to ask how many health interests are operat-ing in the fifty state capitals and what kinds of interests are there. Perhaps it was the case that there were fewer health care interests proportionate to other interests lobbying in state capitals than in the nation's capital in the 1990s, thus making it easier to overcome their opposition and to enact health care reform legislation of all sorts.

Comparison of Federal and State Health Care Interests, 1996–97

As a point of comparison, we use data from the 1996 federal Lobbying Disclosure Reports collected by Frank Baumgartner and Beth Leech to com-pare with lobby registration data we gathered from state legislatures in 1997.[13] Table 1.1 shows the national interest organizations recoded to fit the twenty-six standard categories we use in our research. The categories are ranked by

Table 1.1 National Lobbying Organizations, 1996, Compared with State Lobbying Organizations, 1997

Sector	National Number	National Percent	National Rank	State Number	State Percent	State Rank
Health care practices, disease	739	13.3	1	5,842	16.3	1
Manufacturing	352	6.3	6	3,088	8.6	2
Banking, finance, real estate	442	8.0	2	2,303	6.4	3
Service, other firms	201	3.6	13	2,260	6.3	4
Small business concerns, retailing	94	1.7	17	2,141	6.0	5
Education	339	6.1	8	2,117	5.9	6
Insurance	83	1.5	19	2,058	5.8	7
Government and intergovernmental relations	399	7.2	3	1,517	4.2	8
Human resource issues, welfare services	127	2.3	14	1,395	3.9	9
Communications and media	318	5.7	10	1,345	3.8	10
Utilities and energy generation	221	4.0	12	1,285	3.6	11
Commercial resource development	108	2.0	16	1,256	3.5	12
Sports, amusements, and clubs	65	1.2	20	1,252	3.5	13
Transportation companies and transit issues	322	5.8	9	1,058	3.0	14
Construction, housing	90	1.6	18	1,029	2.9	15
Legal practice and issues, courts	47	0.9	22	841	2.4	16
Agriculture, fisheries	372	6.7	4	838	2.3	17
Police, fire, emergency medical, and corrections	17	0.3	25	796	2.2	18
Environmental preservation, conservation	349	6.3	7	638	1.8	19
Hotel, restaurant, and liquor issues	52	0.9	21	507	1.4	20
Good government and policy advocacy	366	6.6	5	448	1.3	21
Women's issues and abortion	17	0.3	26	321	0.9	22
Taxation issues and governmental regulation	18	0.3	24	317	0.9	23
Civil rights, minority issues	125	2.3	15	241	0.7	24
Religious organizations and churches	19	0.3	23	231	0.7	25
Military and veterans	268	4.8	11	113	0.3	26
Unknown				528	1.5	
Total	5,550	100.0		35,765	100.0	

Note: Health product and pharmaceutical manufacturers are coded under "health" at both the state and national levels.
Sources: For federal agencies, Baumgartner and Leech (1996). For state agencies, lobbying registries of individual states. The data were already coded from prior research by Gray and Lowery.

their frequency at the state level (see the table's far right-hand column for their rank).[14] The reader will note that health care was the largest category of interest organizations at the national level, comprising 13.3 percent of all organizations lobbying in Congress. But the reader may be surprised that health care was an even larger interest category at the state level, comprising 16.3 percent of all interests in the state capitals. Thus it would seem that health reform in the states has been achieved "against all odds," that is, in spite of a substantial lineup of health industry groups. There are even more organized interests, proportionately, to overcome at the state level than at the national level in order to achieve health care reform. Interestingly, our data show that the health category was among those growing the fastest at the state level in the 1990s; between 1990 and 1997, health lobby registrations in state capitals increased 48.8 percent (Gray and Lowery 2001, 268). Only the categories of communications and business services grew faster during the 1990s.

Moreover, health interests are not concentrated in any one state; doctors, nurses, psychologists, optometrists, and other health professionals are organized in every state, as are other health care providers such as hospitals and nursing homes. The same is true for the lobbyists who represent the health insurance and pharmaceutical industries. For example, in our 1997 data set, the Pharmaceutical Research and Manufacturers of America was registered in forty-four states, the Health Insurance Association of America in forty-three states, Pfizer in forty-one states, Pharmacia and Upjohn in forty-one states, and Blue Cross/Blue Shield in forty states. Thus, the same forces that defeat or drastically change some proposals in Washington also operate in state capitals, presumably with financial resources of the same relative magnitude. And theoretically at least, one might think that industry groups would have even greater leverage at the state level than at the national level due to the threat of "exit"; that is, insurers can threaten to leave if they are overregulated or doctors can leave if their malpractice payments are too high. But as we pointed out above, reform happened sooner in the states than in Washington. How has this puzzling situation come about?

We can answer this question only by studying reform where it did happen first—in the states. The health reforms we study in this book occurred in most states but not all, so we are able to exploit this variation among states in the extent of reform and the variation among states in the structure of their organized interest communities, as well as in other key features. Scholars who offer interest-based or institutionally based explanations for the failure of health reforms in Washington cannot systematically test their explanations because they do not have this kind of variation in interest group systems or in institutions. We argue in this section, and at greater length in chapter 2, that health care reforms, like other public policy outcomes, depend upon the structure of the interest group system in each state, particularly its *density* and *diversity*. We have developed a theoretical model of interest system density—the Energy Stability Area (ESA) Model—that we use to examine variations in both the overall size of state interest communities and variations among its categories or sectors of interest organizations, such as provider organizations, insurers, and professional organizations.

We are also interested in the *diversity* of interest communities, that is, in the balance of different types of interest organizations. Unlike density, interest communities can be diverse with respect to any number of traits of interest organizations. Still, most studies of diversity address the balance of the substantive interests represented by organizations, such as those presented already in table 1.1, which shows that health care is especially well represented by lobbying organizations. The most common normative question addressed is whether business interests are too well represented and if their influence might be mitigated by more citizens' groups or groups representing social concerns (Schlozman and Tierney 1986). Although we cannot answer the question of whether business interests overall have too many lobbying representatives, we can compare the national and state interest systems with respect to how well business is represented. Table 1.2 reorganizes our federal and state data so that we can make this comparison. It is clear that business is well represented by lobbying organizations at both levels of governments; for-profit organizations dominate not-for-profit organizations at both levels of government in lobby registrations in 1996 and 1997. However, the for-profit business sector is even better represented at the state level than at the federal level; interest organizations representing businesses were 73.8 percent of the lobby registration at the state level in 1997, whereas they were 62 percent at the federal level in 1996. The high representation of for-profit interests at the state level would seem to operate against successful state reform of the health care system because business was one of the main opponents of federal health care reform.[15] So states have achieved reform in spite of less diversity and a higher concentration of for-profit interest organizations than the national level. Thus, from the standpoint of the state interest group system's density and diversity, health care reformers' prospects were better, on average, in the nation's capital than in the typical state capital. The fact that any health reform legislation has been enacted at all by the states is indeed a story worth investigating and telling.

Table 1.2 Profit and Nonprofit Lobbying Organizations at the State (1997) and National (1996) Levels

Sector	National Number	National Percent	State Number	State Percent
Profit				
Health care practices, delivery, disease	739	13.3	5,842	16.3
Manufacturing	352	6.3	3,088	8.6
Banking, finance, real estate	442	8.0	2,303	6.4
Service, other firms	201	3.6	2,260	6.3
Small business concerns, retailing	94	1.7	2,141	6.0
Insurance	83	1.5	2,058	5.8
Communications and media	318	5.7	1,345	3.8
Utilities and energy generation	221	4.0	1,285	3.6
Commercial resource development	108	2.0	1,256	3.5
Transportation companies and transit issues	322	5.8	1,058	3.0
Construction, housing	90	1.6	1,029	2.9
Legal practice and issues, courts	47	0.9	841	2.4
Agriculture, fisheries	372	6.7	838	2.3
Hotel, restaurant, and liquor issues	52	0.9	507	1.4
Unknown			528	1.5
Subtotal	3,441	62.0	26,379	73.8
Not-for-Profit				
Social	1,227	22.1	3,561	10.0
Sports, amusements, and clubs	65	1.2	1,252	3.5
Environmental preservation, conservation	349	6.3	638	1.8
Good government and policy advocacy	366	6.6	448	1.3
Women's issues and abortion	17	0.3	321	0.9
Taxation issues and governmental regulation	18	0.3	317	0.9
Civil rights, minority issues	125	2.3	241	0.7
Religious organizations and churches	19	0.3	231	0.7
Military and veterans	268	4.8	113	0.3
Government	416	7.5	2,313	6.5
Government and intergovernmental relations	399	7.2	1,517	4.2
Police, fire, emergency medical, and corrections	17	0.3	796	2.2
Education	339	6.1	2,117	5.9
Human resource issues, welfare services	127	2.3	1,395	3.9
Subtotal	2,109	38.0	9,386	26.2
Total	5,550	100.0	35,765	100.0

Note: Health product and pharmaceutical manufacturers are coded under "health" at both the state and national levels.

Sources: For federal agencies, Baumgartner and Leech (1996). For state agencies, lobbying registries of individual states. The data were already coded from prior research by Gray and Lowery.

Our theory of diversity, which is developed in chapter 2, is partly based on the densities of different types of interest organizations, but it is also based on the reaction functions of different interest categories. Health care, just to preview our ESA model, is highly sensitive to changes in the size of the economy and the population. Thus, as states' economies grow, their interest communities will have relatively more organizations representing health care interests.

Configuration of Interests

What pattern of organized interests should we expect to be associated with the adoption of health care reforms? The literature provides at least two sharply competing assessments of the impact of the density and diversity of interest communities on public policy in general (Lowery and Brasher 2004). To some, the presence of large numbers of business interests is sufficient evidence that business must exercise undue influence (Schattschneider 1960; Schlozman and Tierney 1986). But other scholars argue that excessive presence within an interest system represents weakness rather than strength. That is, some core interest must be threatened before it willingly incurs the costs of lobbying (Heinz et al. 1993). Still others suggest that whether the density and diversity of an interest system indicates policy dominance or weakness depends on both the unity of the interest community and the unity and direction of public opinion (Smith 2000). Indeed, the literature on state public policy overall offers mixed findings on the influence of organized interests.

In terms of organized interests' impact on health care policy, Barrilleaux and Miller (1988) reported that the diversity of the interest system was positively associated with Medicaid effort, defined as the proportion of total state personal income spent on Medicaid vendor payments (minus the federal share of Medicaid payments). Grogan (1994), using Gray and Lowery's (1996) 1990 lobby registration data, found that interest pressure affected state Medicaid policy decisions. And Miller (2005), in a meta-analysis of the health policy literature, reported that significant positive results were found for advocacy organizations but rarely existed for provider organizations. Given these findings for the influence of health interest organizations, it seems plausible to expect that the density and diversity of health interest communities in the states might well influence their adoption of new health care policies and their stringency of regulation. We focus on three sets of interests in the models used in our empirical chapters.

The first set is indicators of the organized interest advocates for each of the policy reforms under study. Based on previous studies and newspaper coverage, it is fairly clear which groups supported each of the three reforms; we expect that where there are more interest groups supporting a reform, it is more likely to be adopted. Similarly, if the reform is a regulation, it is likely to be more stringent or if it is a spending program, more generous, where there are more advocates lobbying for it. Among the relevant health policy studies is Pracht and Moore's (2003) analysis of organized interests and pharmacy reimbursement rates in state Medicaid programs. They reported that the rate of participation of pharmacists in state affiliates of the American Pharmaceutical Association was positively associated with Medicaid pharmacy reimbursement rates. We interpret this study as reinforcing our view that the density of health advocacy community increases the likelihood of health reform.

The second set of interest measures consists of the organized interest opponents of each of the policy reforms studied here. Too often, research studies are satisfied with measuring the existence or strength of the supporting coalition without putting effort into measuring the interest organizations on the other side. This is not satisfactory because policy outcomes are the result of the balance of interest group forces; the outcomes are not determined just by what protagonists on one side of an issue do. Baumgartner and colleagues' (2009) study of Washington lobbying on 100 issues demonstrated this point very persuasively; 63 percent of advocates challenging the status quo expected active opposition from organized interests, but even more—86 percent—of those defending the status quo anticipated active opposition from interest groups (Baumgartner, Gray, and Lowery 2009, 79). Thus measurement of the forces on both sides of the issue is critical. Our data set allows us to measure the density of the opponents of each reform as well as its proponents. Miller (2006, 141) is one of the few health policy researchers who have included measures of organized interest opponents in his studies. In an analysis of changes in nursing home reimbursement rates under the Medicaid program, he showed that states with more powerful organized interests representing the elderly and nursing homes were less likely to adopt cost-containing changes. We interpret these studies as consistent with our perspective that the density of organized interest opposition will deter health reform in the states.

The third set of measures to be included in our models is the overall number/proportion of health interests. Given Gray and Lowery's (1995b) finding that crowded interest systems make the passage of *any* legislation more difficult as well as other analyses of policy gridlock, we must account for the effect of crowding. The general policy literature finds that policy agendas are limited (Jones and Baumgartner 2005); the more crowded the agenda, all other things being equal, the less likely that a measure will pass. Moreover, the size of the state interest community is directly and positively responsive to how crowded state policy agendas are (Gray et al. 2005a). Given these complex relationships, we need to control for the density of the interest community and/or the overall proportion of health interest organizations in state interest communities. Finally, we interpret the gridlock literature as saying that health reform is more likely to pass on a less crowded agenda.

Health Reforms as Policy Innovations

The major contribution of this book lies in the policy reforms we examine and our measures of the density and diversity of interest communities. But the interest group measures must of course be embedded in some model of the policymaking process because interest groups are not the only political force at work. Given that we are examining reforms, the additional hypotheses we develop are from research on policy innovation. A policy innovation is simply a "program or policy which is new to the states adopting it, no matter how old the program may be or how many other states may have adopted it" (Walker 1969, 881). The health reforms we study here—state pharmacy assistance programs, antimanaged care regulations, and universal coverage programs—meet this criterion in that they were new to the adopting states, and in addition, the state adoptions preceded enactment by the federal government. Social scientists have studied the diffusion of innovations across time and space since at least 1940 (McVoy 1940). Beginning in the early 1960s, Everett Rogers has compiled research on the topic in his volume *Diffusion of Innovations*. His fifth edition, in 2003, referenced more than 5,200 publications on the topic (Rogers 2003). In political science, Jack Walker Jr. (1969) and Virginia Gray (1973) were the first to study how policy innovations diffused across states. Eventually two contrasting approaches to state innovation research developed, and ultimately there was a synthesis. The first approach focused on a set of *internal determinants* that lead policymakers to adopt a new policy, including state fiscal capacity, short-term economic conditions, interparty competition, election cycles, party control, level of education of the population, legislative professionalism, political culture, strength of organized interests, and public opinion. These are often derived from Lawrence Mohr's (1969, 114) claim that innovation is "directly related to the motivation to innovate, inversely related to the strength of obstacles to innovation, and directly related to the availability of resources for overcoming such obstacles." States with close interparty competition, liberal public opinion, above-average wealth, and under Democratic Party control are thought to have the resources to be more innovative than other states, assuming the innovation is expanding the scope of government. This emphasis on the internal characteristics of states continues in the most recent scholarship. For example, Boushey (2010), in one of the recent full-scale treatments of the dynamics of policy diffusion, argues that states are more or less receptive to different kinds of innovation due to their political, institutional, and socioeconomic characteristics.

A second tradition focused on *external forces* leading states to adopt new policies, including the use of a successful policy by neighboring states or ideologically similar states (Grossback, Nicholson-Crotty, and Peterson 2004), or reaction to competing states, emulation of national leader states, influence of professional networks, and in response to financial incentives or disincentives provided by the federal government or national media salience (Karch 2007). Boushey (2010, 20–21) argues that interest groups, policy activists, and policy entrepreneurs significantly shape diffusion dynamics across state lines. Another recent article (Pacheco 2012) argues that even ordinary citizens get involved by learning about neighboring policies and changing their own opinions on policies. If state opinion becomes positive, then responsive state officials will enact similar policies in the home state. By far, the most studied external influence is regional diffusion or the impact of neighbors' policies. For some policies—the lottery, for example—regional diffusion is quite plausible (Berry and Berry 1990). Moreover, regional diffusion is more easily studied than other types of diffusion. Emulation of neighboring states can reduce the perceived risks of policy adoption, thereby producing the political will to overcome obstacles to innovation.

Contemporary scholarship tends to draw upon both approaches with empirical models containing measures of a state's social, political, and economic characteristics as well as its external environment, such as the adoption history of its neighbors (e.g., Berry and Berry 1990; Mintrom 1997). Boushey (2012) has introduced the Bass mixed influence diffusion model as a way of distinguishing external and internal influences on diffusion of innovations. We draw upon the innovation literature for theoretical background to inform our study of the adoption of the three sets of health policy reforms.

Framing explanations of health policy reforms as policy innovations that might diffuse across states is less common in the health policy literature than in the political science literature. A few examples of treating health reforms as policy innovations do stand out, however. Balla (2001) posited that interstate professional associations are the mechanisms by which innovations are diffused. In support of his claim, he found that states whose insurance commissioners participated in the National Association of Insurance Commissioners were more likely to adopt the HMO Model Act. Volden (2006) hypothesized that state leaders emulate successful programs in other states, and he demonstrated this effect in his analysis of success in the CHIP program. Karch (2007) expanded the focus from simple adoption of an innovation to policy content and examined the impact of what he calls "national intervention," a measure of issue salience. He applied his ideas successfully to two health reforms—state pharmacy assistance programs and medical savings accounts—and three welfare programs. Esterling (2009) analyzed a problem in bottom-up vertical diffusion (from the states to the federal government). He posits that federal decision makers will take state expertise more seriously if state and national policy interests are aligned. He demonstrates that state testimony is taken more seriously in Medicare hearings (where interests are aligned) than in Medicaid hearings (where interests are in conflict), thus limiting the value of the states as "laboratories of democracy" that should benefit one another and the federal government. Satterthwaite (2002) has a more explicit intent: to explain the diffusion of managed care in the Medicaid program. He finds that states are more likely to adopt managed care if they are wealthy, have a long history with HMOs, and have neighbors who have adopted. Finally, Miller (2006) contrasts the factors that lead states to adopt innovations in Medicaid nursing facility reimbursement policy versus those that lead them to make only incremental changes in reimbursement policy. He finds that strong governing capacity is an explanation for policy adoption but not for incremental change.

Internal Determinants of Innovation in Our Models

Our first task is to explicate the factors within a state that make it more likely to adopt a new program in health policy, aside from the interest group configuration. We think the most important factors are the problem environment for health care, the resources available to handle the problem, and the political will that exists to attack the problem.

THE PROBLEM ENVIRONMENT

The problem environment is generally regarded as an impetus for policymakers to seek out new policy solutions (Nice 1994). It may be a crisis, a focusing event, or a triggering event (see Birkland 2006)—such as the September 11, 2001, terrorist attacks—that compels action, or it may be a budget shortfall that demonstrates that indeed "necessity is the mother of invention." Or it may be a gap between expectations and results that leads policymakers to adopt a new approach to solving the problem. President George Bush's No Child Left Behind Act of 2001 is an example of the latter. The president believed that the results of elementary and high school education were not satisfactory, so he urged a new federal approach. Problem environment and problem recognition affect innovation in several ways. They bring attention to new issues and thereby force them onto the already-crowded policy agenda; they motivate policymakers to engage in a search for better solutions to existing problems; and under certain conditions they may bring major change.

Problem severity/need stands out as an important stimulus for the adoption of innovation (Sapat 2004; Nice 1994) and as an influence on state regulatory effort (Lester et al. 1983) in the general state politics literature. In the health care arena, Yackee (2009) has demonstrated the impact of a problem severity on medical malpractice reform, Barrilleaux and Brace (2007) its impact on the adoption of policies to promote access to health care, and Pracht (2007) its impact on capitated managed care enrollment in Medicaid. In health care the problems commonly identified at the state level in the 1990s were a lack of access to health care, the costs of health care (including costs of prescription drugs), and complaints about managed care. For example, escalating health care costs were a key "crisis" motivating states to adopt universal coverage (Paul-Shaheen 1998) and pharmacy assistance programs for seniors (Reforming States Group 2003). Of particular importance, the severity of these problems varied across the states, which offered us considerable interstate variation to analyze. This book's empirical chapters present major reforms that states adopted in the 1990s (and earlier) to solve such problems, and in each chapter we present a model that incorporates measures of problem severity that are hypothesized to indicate the need for the reform.

Market structure is the second environmental condition included in our health innovation models. In deciding how to handle severe health care problems, state policymakers confronted a variety of market conditions. Some policymakers faced traditional fee-for-service markets; some confronted highly competitive managed care markets; and others found the state divided into diverse markets, depending upon their urban or rural composition. So just as other health policy researchers control for nursing home bed supply or physician supply, we control for managed care market penetration in our models. We have different expectations about the effect of HMO penetration in our models, depending upon which of the three innovations we are addressing. HMOs were at one time viewed positively as the solution to the crisis in health costs because of their ability to manage costs, but their very success in this regard led to consumer backlash against "rationing" and the subsequent calls for state regulations. The former perspective would indicate a negative coefficient for some of our re-

YBP Library Services

GRAY, VIRGINIA, 1945-

INTEREST GROUPS AND HEALTH CARE REFORM ACROSS THE
UNITED STATES.
                              Paper   336 P.
WASHINGTON: GEORGETOWN UNIV PRESS, 2013
SER: AMERICAN GOVERNANCE AND PUBLIC POLICY.

AUTH: UNIVERSITY OF NORTH CAROLINA, CHAPEL HILL.
ASSESSES IMPACT OF GROUPS IN SHAPING POLICY.
LCCN 2012-37462
  ISBN 158901989X   **Library PO#** FIRM ORDERS

		List	29.95	USD
8395 NATIONAL UNIVERSITY LIBRAR	**Disc**	5.0%		
App. Date 4/16/14 SHHS 8214-08	**Net**	28.45	USD	

SUBJ: 1. HEALTH CARE REFORM--POL. ASPECTS--U.S.
2. MEDICAL POLICY--U.S.
AWD/REV: 2013 YBPL
CLASS RA395   DEWEY# 362.10425097 LEVEL GEN-AC

YBP Library Services

GRAY, VIRGINIA, 1945-

INTEREST GROUPS AND HEALTH CARE REFORM ACROSS THE
UNITED STATES.
                              Paper   336 P.
WASHINGTON: GEORGETOWN UNIV PRESS, 2013
SER: AMERICAN GOVERNANCE AND PUBLIC POLICY.

AUTH: UNIVERSITY OF NORTH CAROLINA, CHAPEL HILL.
ASSESSES IMPACT OF GROUPS IN SHAPING POLICY.
  LCCN 2012-37462
  ISBN 158901989X   **Library PO#** FIRM ORDERS

		List	29.95	USD
8395 NATIONAL UNIVERSITY LIBRAR	**Disc**	5.0%		
App. Date 4/16/14 SHHS 8214-08	**Net**	28.45	USD	

SUBJ: 1. HEALTH CARE REFORM--POL. ASPECTS--U.S.
2. MEDICAL POLICY--U.S.
AWD/REV: 2013 YBPL
CLASS RA395   DEWEY# 362.10425097 LEVEL GEN-AC

forms, while the latter position suggests a positive coefficient. The latter position has been bolstered by the evidence of Satterthwaite (2002) and Volden (2006). Each of them found that diffusion of different innovations in health policy was influenced positively by the HMO structure of the states.

RESOURCES

Although an excess of problems may provoke officials to act in innovative ways, more often innovation probably results from the richness of resources, argue most scholars of innovation who adhere to the "theory of slack resources" (Walker 1969). The idea here is that bold thinking is more likely to occur when policymakers have the time, expertise, and financial resources to identify problems and search for solutions. A resource-rich environment is more likely to attract skilled professionals interested in innovation, to encourage their visionary thinking, and to have enough uncommitted resources to implement new and experimental programs. Accordingly, affluent states are most likely to have public policy environments supportive of innovation.

State wealth has been a staple concept of innovation studies since the notion was first put forward by Jack Walker in 1969. He described a relationship between wealth, urbanization, industrialization, and the early enactment of policy innovations. Researchers routinely find that wealthier states are more likely to innovate, and we expect the same here for health care reforms. Indeed, Grogan (1993) argued that with respect to health care *only* relatively wealthy states can innovate. Satterthwaite (2002) found that wealthy states were more likely to adopt a managed care model in their Medicaid programs. And Miller (2005) reported in his meta-analysis that wealthier, more economically developed states were more likely to provide the medical services studied. Similarly, the greater the amount of resources available to the state, the more likely the state can afford to undertake more stringent environmental regulation, as demonstrated by Sapat (2004).

State capacity is a related concept that refers to the extent to which the state has deployed its financial resources so as to increase the professionalism of the executive branch, thereby raising the likelihood of innovation. Administrative capacity is presumed to be linked to state wealth, but of course rich states might choose not to spend their resources on the state bureaucracy but elsewhere. Administrative capacity has been shown to be a significant determinant of adopting redistributive health reforms (Barrilleaux and Brace 2007). Moreover, in the literature on the politics of regulation, it is well recognized that enhanced administrative capacity leads to greater independent regulation (Teske 2004). Miller's summary of the health policy literature (2005) indicates that states with greater administrative capacity have more active and influential bureaucracies in state health policymaking.

THE POLITICAL CLIMATE

The political climate or environment within a state greatly affects its likelihood for innovation in various policy areas. Political scientists have used many measures of state politics over the years as correlates of innovation rankings, but three stand out as especially relevant to the process of innovation consideration and adoption in health policy.

Political ideology is a concept capturing the state's relative liberalism or conservatism, that is, its citizens' preferences for a larger or smaller scope of government. It is hypothesized that the general ideological environment of a state influences the probability of a policy innovation being enacted (Grossback, Nicholson-Crotty, and Peterson 2004). In health policy Miller's meta-analysis (2005) discovered that state public opinion was the most frequently studied political determinant. The findings were unequivocal: Liberal public opinion was positively associated with many health policy outcomes. For example, Yackee (2009) found that citizen ideology positively influenced the passage of medical malpractice reforms.

Party control is perhaps the aspect of state political climate most often linked to policy innovation. Depending upon the type of innovation, Republican or Democratic control might be most advantageous. If innovations expand the scope of government by adding new programs or spending more money, then Democratic gubernatorial and legislative control is predicted to be associated. If innovations restrict the scope of government by privatizing services or restricting government growth, then Republican Party control would be expected to be operating. Miller's meta-analysis (2005) of the determinants of public health policy outcomes demonstrated that Democratic governors were more likely to be supportive than Republicans.

Interparty competition is the third internal political concept likely to affect policy innovation. As far back as Walker (1969), it was argued that a political party facing a closely contested election would try to outdo the other party by advocating the newest programs. Thus, states with higher levels of interparty competition would over time display higher levels of innovations. As recently as Boushey's (2010) study of innovation receptivity, political competition was among his most significant and substantively highest-impact variables. In the health policy literature, Pracht (2007) discovered that the more evenly competition was divided between the state's two major parties, the more likely it was that its Medicaid plan had embraced the new capitated managed care model.

EXTERNAL DIFFUSION SOURCES

All the factors discussed so far are internal to the state, but researchers also assume that forces external to the state influence its proclivity to adopt new ideas. Developments elsewhere, especially successful ones, come to the attention of state legislators and state bureaucrats through professional networks and associations. Or national debate and media activity can increase an issue's salience so that state legislators can no longer ignore the issue (Karch 2007). The federal government may provide financial incentives or disincentives that affect the pace of adoption of innovations (Welch and Thompson 1980). And the fact that a state's neighbors have already adopted a policy often increases the likelihood of adoption, for example, the lottery spread through regional diffusion (Berry and Berry 1990). In sum, state policymakers do not reinvent the wheel when faced with a new problem; they often turn to a state or states that have already solved the problem and imitate their policy.

HORIZONTAL DIFFUSION

Horizontal diffusion is by far the most studied type of diffusion, that is, from one state to another. Various researchers, from Walker (1969) to Canon and Baum (1981) to Berry and Berry (1992), have found regional diffusion effects to be important in explaining the spread of policy innovations (for a literature review, see Miller 2004). Most researchers focus on neighboring or contiguous states, theorizing that policymakers pay closest attention to what is going on in bordering states or in other nearby states because they have similar problems. However, Walker's seminal article (1969) also called attention to "leader states" such as California and New York that many states around the country like to emulate and to the idea that a state can be a regional leader for a smaller group of states. Gray (1973) developed the notion that such reference groups vary by issue area, that is, the leader states in health care are not the same as the leader states in corrections policy. In the health arena, Miller (2006), Grogan (1994), Kim and Jennings (2012), and Satterthwaite (2002) confirmed that regional diffusion explained changes in different parts of the Medicaid program. Yackee (2009) found regional diffusion effects to be important for the diffusion of medical malpractice reform, while Balla (2001) found diffusion from geographic neighbors and interstate associational ties both explained the diffusion pattern of the model HMO Act. Accordingly, we include a measure of neighboring states' policy activity in our models.

VERTICAL DIFFUSION: TOP-DOWN

Vertical diffusion usually describes a top-down process, whereby national influences—such as the federal government, national professional associations, the media, and other national external influences—make an impact on the spread of innovations across states. Vertical diffusion can also be a bottom-up process, whereby the states influence the federal government. The federal government's top-down effects have been thoroughly documented, starting with Gray's 1973 article, which demonstrated that federal grant money speeds up the spread of innovations (Gray 1973). By offering financial incentives, the federal government can encourage policies to diffuse more rapidly and to be adopted by more states than would otherwise be the case (Allen, Pettus, and Haider-Markel 2004). And it is not just federal dollars that matter; federal mandates matter as well. Shipan and Volden (2006), for example, showed that the passage of federal legislation preventing the sale of cigarettes to underage youth had a strong positive effect upon state adoption of youth access laws, even alongside the presence of a regional diffusion effect. In another example of vertical diffusion, Kim and Jennings (2012) demonstrated that the federal Balanced Budget Act in 1997, with its greater waiver flexibility for states in their Medicaid programs, contributed to an 8.7 percent increase in managed-care enrollment in that program. And the failure of the national government to take action in a policy domain, perhaps due to divided government, can itself be an impetus for state policymakers to act themselves (Allen, Pettus, and Haider-Markel 2004). The strength of the signal from the federal government can mobilize interest groups to take their battle to the state level, depending upon whether the groups represent the opponents or proponents of the policy action.

National political developments, whether they succeed in the enactment of federal legislation or not, are another external force capable of affecting state political agendas (Baumgartner, Gray, and Lowery 2009). Clearly, the two-year-long debate over President Clinton's Health Security Plan in 1993–94 put universal coverage prominently on the national agenda, and its failure removed the possibility from the federal agenda for more than a decade. However, as we show in chapter 5, universal coverage moved to the state level, where nearly all states considered it, and quite a few enacted some version of it, albeit on an experimental basis. In a different case, thirty-four states had quietly covered the pharmaceutical needs of senior citizens with their own assistance programs while Congress did nothing. Finally, in his 1999 State of the Union Address, President Clinton put senior drug coverage on the national agenda when he proposed adding a new drug benefit to Medicare. This focused public attention on the issue, which led both presidential candidates—George W. Bush and Al Gore—to offer plans for Medicare reform during the 2000 campaign. Part D was eventually added to Medicare in 2003 under President Bush.

Andrew Karch (2007), in a pathbreaking study of five health and welfare innovations, argued that national policy developments are an influential external source and that newspaper coverage of issues is a good proxy for the visibility of national policy developments. Time-pressed state officials turn to these cues or examples. For national activity to influence state policymaking, it must be visible and politically salient to people at the state level. And national developments must precede state-level activity in order to have a causal impact on the states, he argues. Scott Lamothe (2003) had developed a similar argument about external influence through the mass media, measured by a citation count; however, he reasoned that media attention would have the most impact on state legislators in the year of enactment. Finally, Nicholson-Crotty (2009) has demonstrated that high salience–low complexity policies are likely to diffuse more rapidly than other types of policies. We will follow the lead of these researchers and develop a media coverage index for each policy innovation we study.

Vertical Diffusion: Bottom-Up

Vertical diffusion can also refer to the bottom-up process whereby the states are the "laboratories of democracy" for the national government, with policies being tested first at the state level and then being adopted by the national government. The evidence for the occurrence of this process is more limited, usually based on studies of a small number of state policy experiments, such as a study by Boeckelman (1992) of redistributive policy and by Arsneault (2000) on welfare policy. Of most direct relevance to this project is Weissert and Scheller's analysis (2008) of six federal enactments in health policy that had intergovernmental impacts. They found policy learning in only two of the six examples—CHIP and HIPAA—where state experience was extensive, strong state lobbies existed, and federal government expertise was very low or non-existent. In the other four cases, state experience was largely ignored. Finally, in one of the most extensive tests of the bottom-up thesis, Lowery, Gray, and Baumgartner (2011) found little evidence that changes in state policy agendas in the aggregate influenced national patterns of policy attention. In this project, we discuss bottom-up diffusion where we think it occurred, but we do not have a formal test for it.

Policy Content and Process as Innovation

Finally, our examination of each health policy reform goes beyond the adoption of the policy to consider the policy's content: what is being diffused from state to state. Boushey (2010) in particular has argued that the content or characteristics of innovations possess attributes that make them susceptible to incremental diffusion or to policy outbreaks. Others, such as Volden (2006), have argued for an expanded focus on policy content, specifically on states' revision of or amendments to the initial innovation. He discovered that states learned from the success of other states, particularly in lowering the costs of the CHIP program. Previous researchers had considered any changes during the policy adoption process to be *reinvention* and had found that policies adopted later were often more expansive than those adopted earlier, though no theoretical basis was given for this finding (Glick and Hays 1991, 842; Hays 1996; Boehmke and Witmer 2004; Stream 1999). However, Kim and Jennings (2012) found just the opposite: Later adopters of Medicaid managed care programs tended to implement less extensive programs than earlier adopters, controlling for other factors. We examine the revision and generosity of state pharmacy assistance programs, the stringency of anti-HMO regulations, and the type and scope of universal coverage laws under consideration by states. Although the adoption of a new policy remains the most common measure of state policy innovation, we go beyond that to more refined measures.

Other scholars, such as Karch (2007), have argued for a focus on the process of innovation, specifically on the agenda-setting stage, not just the enactment stage. Karch (2007), like Mintrom (1997) before him, used separate explanatory models for the legislative consideration stage and the enactment stage. Karch believes that state legislators import templates of programs from other states and then proceed to customize the templates for their own states, guided by electoral considerations. Lobbying and political action committee contributions are critical components in the customization phase. Our examination of revision and generosity in one program, stringency of regulations in another, and type and scope of coverage in a third program demonstrates our commitment to learning about policy content, not just adoption, and learning about the process of innovation beyond the initial adoption.

Design of the Study

We have touted the analytic benefits of studying health reforms at the state level due to the leverage of variation encountered among the fifty states in the extent of reform and the variation on the explanatory variables, whether they are variations in interest group configuration, problem environment, resources, or political context. These are analytic benefits not available at the national level. However, we do need to set some parameters on our study if it is to be a state-level study and not an intergovernmental study. Accordingly, we have purposefully chosen three important state health reforms that were undertaken with state funds only; we do not study other programs that were jointly funded by the states and the federal government, such as CHIP and Medicaid. As Barrilleaux and Brace (2007, 662) note, policies funded solely from state coffers are the products of different politics than policies that receive national government funds. If we had chosen to study intergovernmental health programs, then clearly we would have needed a model of intergovernmental policymaking that included interest group variables from both levels of government, political and resource measures from both levels, and some account of their interaction over a long period. The specification of such a model would be very complicated. Indeed, the literature does not have well-established or widely accepted models of such vertical diffusion processes. Nor is it our purpose to invent one here.

More to the point, we have noted that our analytic purpose lies in assessing the role of organized interests in public policy with a secondary interest in understanding variation in the adoption of state health policies. By delimiting the analysis to state policies on which the states are fully responsible for adoption and implementation, we control for a number of confounding variables, especially those associated with vertical diffusion from the federal government. If our purpose is to explain how organized interests influence state policy adoption, then we can best accomplish that by analyzing state-level models. Of course, consistent with innovation theory, we examine horizontal and vertical sources of diffusion. But the point is that by analyzing state-funded programs, we keep the impact of the latter at a minimum. In each of the empirical chapters (3, 4, and 5), we describe the specific health reforms, their history, and the specific measures used in the general model outlined in this chapter.

Conclusion

This concludes our exposition of policy innovation theory and its application to our three cases, which have been discussed briefly. In addition, this chapter has introduced the critical role of organized interests in shaping or blocking the passage of health care legislation, the central purpose of our analysis, and a topic we consider much more thoroughly in the discussion of the following chapters on specific proposed reforms. This chapter has also brought us up to date on how the ACA of 2010 may have an impact on the states. We compared the density and diversity of health organizations at the state and national levels in order to make the point that health care reformers face similar interest configurations at both levels of government. Next, we presented the major concepts to be used in the empirical analyses in chapters 3, 4, and 5. The following chapter presents more data on the structure of health interest communities in the fifty states and explicates our ecological theory about the density and diversity of organized interests.

Together, these elements should provide a firm foundation to provide a better, more persuasive, and perhaps more useful assessment of the role of organized interests in American politics. As we noted in the introduction of this chapter, scholarship, journalism, and the daily complaints of citizens offer such widely divergent views of the role of organized interests in American politics that even the most simple facts, such as very presence of large numbers of business interests in lobbying communities, often lead to conclusions about influence as different as black and white. With attention to the actual patterns of adoption across the fifty states of several different policies of considerable variation in scope, salience, and incidence in terms of how they bear on different interests, we hope to provide a more valid assessment of when and how organized interests influence public policy.

Notes

1. CHIP was enacted in the wake of the failure of Clinton's plan for universal access; though it helps the states insure low-income children modestly above the Medicaid limit, it leaves many other children uninsured. The Medicaid 1115 waiver program allows states to seek approval for demonstration projects that would run afoul of existing Medicaid policy. Examples are putting patients into managed care, "cash and counseling," and responding to Hurricane Katrina (Thompson and Burke 2007). But while such waivers support bottom-up innovation, they are supposed to be budget neutral to the federal government. Thompson and Burke (2007, 988–89) conclude that "clearly, 1115 waivers have not succeeded in galvanizing universal coverage in particular states. . . . In a more incremental way, however, many of the waivers bolstered access to health services for low-income people." They also find it striking that even President George W. Bush was not able to use these waivers as a major tool for Medicaid program erosion. But overall these waivers were not a major solution to the problem of the uninsured and their lack of access to health care.

2. The decision was actually a set of decisions in three related cases: *National Federation of Independent Business et al. v. Sebelius*, No. 11-393; *Department of Health and Human Services v. Florida et al.*, No. 11-398; and *Florida et al. v. Department of Health and Human Services*, No. 11-400.

3. Jacobs (2011) has also relied on path dependency theory to describe the passage of the ACA as a critical juncture which will trigger a new developmental path in health policy (see also Haeder [2012] for a discussion of path dependency as an explanation for the passage of the ACA and see Brown [2010] for an argument against the use of path dependence in health policy).

4. A study by Center for Responsive Politics (2010) sought to determine why there has been an overall decline in the number of registered lobbyists and groups since the Honest Leadership and Open Government Act (HLOGA) went into effect in 2008 and since President Obama took office in January 2009, putting several antilobbyist initiatives into effect. The Center for Responsive Politics determined that most lobby deregistrations occurred in 2008, the year HLOGA went into effect, rather than in 2009, after President Obama came into office.

5. For details on the effects of the "doughnut hole," see Rosenthal (2004).

6. This was as of April 1, 2010.

7. Nineteen states operate programs that negotiate discounts on drug prices with pharmaceutical companies on behalf of eligible citizens, as of April 1, 2010; these programs do not cost states money. Some states offer both programs.

8. For example, in 2001 the interstate mobility rate of the population over 62 with incomes up to 200 percent above the poverty line was 5.8 percent, as compared with the 12.4 percent mobility rate of the total population. With a mobility rate less than half that of the general population, it hardly suggests that seniors are moving across state lines for help with their drug bills, as compared with favorable rates on income and sales taxes and capital gains and proximity to the grandkids.

9. A single-payer plan is a government-administered health plan with no involvement from private insurers.

10. We use the acronym "ACA" to refer to the 2010 law rather than the term "Obamacare," which was used as a term of derision during the congressional battle of 2009–10.

11. One new federal agency was created within the Department of Health and Human Services—the Office of Consumer Information and Insurance Oversight. It implements many of the legislative provisions that address private health insurance and thus will work closely with the states.

12. These pools, to be used only until 2014, could build upon those already existing in thirty states and will receive federal financial support; or states can let the Department of Health and Human Services do it alone.

13. The 1996 data are the first federal data available since the passage of the 1995 Lobbying Disclosure Act. No such data were available during the years 1993–94.

14. The percentages here may differ from ones previously published by Virginia Gray and David Lowery because health products and pharmaceutical manufacturers are coded here under health rather than under manufacturing, as was done in some early articles.

15. For example, in the 2009–10 health reform fight, the business community overall, with the exception of Wal-Mart, opposed a mandate on employers to provide insurance to all employees; they lobbied heavily and successfully to convert play or pay to a tax on large employers for not playing and a subsidy for small businesses to play.

CHAPTER 2

The Theory and Structure of Health Interest Communities in the States

Politicians, media commentators, and scholars alike long have been concerned about the role of organized interests in public policy. Of particular concern is the seeming dominance of business over citizens and not-for-profit groups. In spite of this concern about the balance of different types of interest organizations in the population as a whole, the conversation in much of the media is about individual interest organizations. How is a given firm or association mobilized? What actions has it undertaken to influence public officials? And how influential is it? But there are limits to what we can learn by looking at one or a few interest organizations. Simply put, public policy is influenced by all of their actions in combination. Although we will see that some subsets of the interest population are at times more influential than others, we cannot get a comprehensive understanding of their overall influence on policy unless we address the full population of interests that might be engaged in influencing a related set of public policies.

Within the past decade, the importance of a population-level focus fully emerged as political researchers and practitioners realized that features of an interest organization community—the balance of allied and opposed organizations, short-term coalitions of organizations, and competition between similar organizations, just to name a few—have a direct bearing on the organizational health, strategic behavior, and success of individual interest organizations (e.g., Nownes 2000; Nownes and Lapinski 2005; Baumgartner, Gray and Lowery 2009; Halpin and Jordan 2009; Messer, Berkhout, and Lowery 2011; Grossman 2012). The objective in this second chapter is to become more familiar with the features of the health interest organization communities in the American states and the theories and concepts that help us to understand their composition. This is a necessary first step in understanding how and why the several different configurations of interest organization communities studied in chapters 3 through 5 are likely to have diverse patterns of influence on health reform policy.

In chapter 2, then, we examine the structure of the health interest organization system in the fifty states using a population ecology approach, specifically, the Energy Stability Area (ESA) model of interest communities introduced in chapter 1. We begin with a brief introduction to the history of scholarship studying interest organizations as communities. We then present our data on the density and diversity of health interest groups operating in state capitals during the 1990s. The density and diversity data are examined in terms of both variation over time and variation across states. Finally, we present data that connect the population of health interest groups lobbying at the state level to the population of political action committees (PACs) operating in the same arena.

The Study of Interest Organization Communities

Scholars have developed three quite different explanations for the growth and composition of interest organization communities. Some provide a far more benign assessment of the effect of large and growing interest communities on policy and governance than others. Two of the three most prominent explanations of the growth of interest communities are firmly rooted in explanations of the mobilization of individual interest organizations. The first explanation was put forth by David Truman in his 1951 book *The Governmental Process*. He argued that interest groups form when like-minded individuals come together to address shared or common problems. In this view, mobilization, or the formation of interest organizations, is a natural and spontaneous response as citizens seek solutions to disturbances in their lives through public policy. To Truman, then, the eventual size of the interest community is limited only by the number and intensity of disturbances giving rise to the mobilization of new interest organizations. With greater social and economic complexity, the number and intensity of disturbances at least potentially amenable to public policy solutions grow. Therefore, if interest communities are becoming ever more crowded, then that is merely the result of a society that is growing increasingly complex. Of particular importance, Truman recognized but did not attend to interest communities per se. In his view all the interesting action occurs at the level of individual interest organizations and how they are mobilized. The interest community is generated merely through the accumulation of these mobilization events. And the size of this community changes with the frequency of disturbances, giving rise to the mobilization or demobilization of individual interest organizations.

The second explanation of the density of interest organization communities, from Mancur Olson, is also firmly rooted in an understanding of how individual interest organizations are created. In his 1965 book *The Logic of Collective Action*, Olson rejected Truman's argument that mobilization was natural. Rather, he argued that individuals have incentives to free ride or to let others address policy issues of concern to them by participating in interest groups. We would benefit from the actions of the groups even without exerting ourselves so long as others did so. But if all individuals make such calculations, then no one will make the effort to form organizations to address shared problems. Thus, shared problems are not enough to ensure mobilization. Indeed, in Olson's view, only certain kinds of interest organizations are likely to form. The first are very small groups where free riding is readily observed and thereby inhibited, especially small groups with large stakes in public policy. Thus, Olson implied that automobile companies will far more readily organize to prevent the adoption of clean air regulations than will citizens concerned about environmental air quality. Second, however, even larger groups can overcome incentives to free ride by providing selective benefits for joining a group. Unlike the collective benefit arising from a public policy solution to a shared disturbance, a selective benefit is received only through membership in the group. Thus, though those concerned with air quality will benefit from pollution regulations whether or not they participate in an environmental group, they cannot receive the environmental organization's magazine or its discounts on hiking trips unless they actually join. Yet, though effective, the use of selective benefits to overcome collective action problems arising from free riding may come at a cost. That is, membership in such organizations may be no longer linked to a policy issue or shared disturbance but may be based instead on receipt of the selective benefit. Thus, according to Olson, any lobbying the organization undertakes is merely a by-product of the provision of selective benefits, not pursuit of collective benefits associated with addressing shared problems.

How then, in Olson's view, are interest organization communities constructed? In one respect, Olson's account of interest organization density is similar to Truman's. That is, interest communities are formed merely through the summation of individual mobilization events. As organized interests discover solutions to collective action problems, the interest community will grow larger. Small groups with large stakes in public policy might organize more readily. But over time, even large groups will join the interest community based on a provision of selective benefits. At this point, however, Olson's analysis of interest communities departs sharply from Truman's by asserting that interest groups rarely die once having overcome free riding. Indeed, Olson concluded that "organizations with selective incentives in stable societies normally survive indefinitely" (Olson 1982, 40). In Olson's analysis, if members join organizations largely for selective benefits, they will remain members even after the policy disturbance initially justifying the group's formation is solved.[1] More to the point, if interest organizations fueled by selective benefits survive indefinitely, then the growth of interest populations is unconstrained. Interest communities will always grow, even until the costs they impose on society through the adoption of policies of special benefit to themselves cause economies to slow and even collapse, a process Olson labeled the institutional sclerosis hypothesis.

Although sharply disagreeing with each other, scholars became increasingly dissatisfied with both of these mobilization-based accounts of the construction of interest communities. Just as Olson's analysis of collective action sharply undermined Truman's assumption that mobilization was natural and inevitable, research on individual motivations for joining interest organizations increasingly showed that Olson's analysis of free riding was at least overstated.[2] These findings have important implications for explaining the density of interest communities by suggesting that the process by which individual mobilization events are summed to form interest communities is far more complex than either Olson or Truman thought. Just as important, empirical examinations of actual populations of interest organizations suggest that something more than just a simple process of accumulation is occurring (Gray and Lowery 1996, 1998a). In short, something more seems to be occurring with populations of organized interests than can be accounted for by examining only the manner in which individual organizations are mobilized.

The third explanation of interest organization community density, the population ecology approach, arose from this dissatisfaction. The most important characteristic of this account of interest community density is its assumption that populations are more than a simple accumulation of mobilization events. These events are clearly important. As organizations form, they become the raw material from which interest communities are sculpted. But the population ecology explanation posits that something unique happens at the population level that does the sculpting. Before examining these population-level processes, however, it is worth noting that this explanation is to at least some extent agnostic about whether Truman's or Olson's view of the mobilization of individual interest organizations is more valid. One version of the population ecology explanation, we will see, borrows insights from Truman's analysis. But the explanatory processes highlighted by the population ecology approach should operate equally well whether mobilization occurs as described by Olson or by Truman.

Rather than starting with mobilization, the population ecology approach highlights the role of environmental resources in constraining the size of organizational populations. That is, organizations are assumed to be dependent upon resources in the environment for their survival. Thus, the relative abundance of these resources largely determines the carrying capacity of the political system for organized interests or how many organizations can survive. In this contest for survival, critically, the most telling kind of competition is among similar organized interests or those that are dependent upon the same kinds of environmental resources.

The Energy Stability Area Model

Gray and Lowery's (1996) ESA model, summarized in table 2.1, is rooted in population biology theories of species that highlight the role of environmental resources in constraining the size of populations, communities, and ecosystems. These constraints are viewed as so severe as to more proximally determine the size and composition of ecological communities. That is, in describing the formation of interest communities, the ESA model is fundamentally a contextual explanation that emphasizes environmental constraints, not individual-level motivations.

Thus, the key variable determining vital rates of interest organizations is the presence of other interest organizations potentially representing the same interest. This variable is the area or supply term of the ESA model, which is usually interpreted as the potential number of constituents in the interest domain that might be represented by an interest organization (e.g., the number of hospitals in the state). The main effect of this variable is expected to be positive, so that we should observe more mobilized organizations when we observe more potential constituents (e.g., the more hospitals, the more organizations to represent hospitals). But this relationship is also expected to be progressively less positive, so that growth rates decline as the numbers of potential constituents increase. This reflects density dependence, or crowding, within the community as more and more nominally similar organizations competitively exclude each other from an ever-finer and more precise representation of the interests and the resources needed to maintain the organizations (e.g., teaching hospitals, Catholic hospitals, nonprofit hospitals, for-profit hospitals, rural hospitals). At some point, quite simply, there will be a declining marginal return from a more fine-grained representation of interests and reliance on an ever-narrower resource base. As a result, and in sharp contrast to Olson's expectations, the birthrates of new organizations should decline and/

Table 2.1 Key Concepts of the ESA Model

Concept	Definition	Example of Indicators
Carrying capacity	The number of interest organizations that a system can sustain given the supply of resources	Maximum number of health interest organizations in a state
Area	The potential number of constituents in the interest domain that might be represented by an interest organization	Number of hospitals that could join state hospital association
Crowding or density dependence	The positive relationship between the number of constituents and the number of interest organizations, up to the point when nominally similar organizations competitively exclude each other from resources	Number of interest organizations squared
Energy	The policy issues of concern to an interest domain and the level of uncertainty surrounding their resolution	Size of the political agenda; party competition
Stability	Absence of stressors, such as wars and revolution	An unmeasured constant for stable, postwar Western democracies
Density	The number of interest organizations in a community	Number of interest organizations registered to lobby a state legislature
Diversity	The balance of different types of interest organizations within a community	Nonprofit vs. for-profit organizations

Source: Constructed by the authors.

or the death rates of older organizations should increase as interest communities become more crowded (Gray and Lowery 2001; Nownes 2004; Nownes and Lipinski 2005).

The energy or demand term in the ESA model refers to whether a government provides goods and services the lobbying organization values and the level of uncertainty about their allocation that are used to stimulate mobilization. These are typically measured by the size of the political agenda in a given policy area and level of party competition, respectively (Gray et al. 2005a; Lowery et al. 2004; Brasher, Lowery, and Gray 1999). Thus, the energy term of the model reflects well Truman's (1951) notion that policy disturbances promote mobilization. In the ESA model, however, this is a more secondary determinant that raises or lowers the more important density response function with respect to area, as described above.

The stability term of the model is a constant in our application to the contemporary American states. But population biology's notion of stability agrees with Olson's insight that interest communities must be largely reconstructed from scratch after profound changes in political regimes, such as after a devastating war. But whereas Olson (1982) viewed such processes as occurring over a century or so, ESA empirical analyses have found that political systems reach equilibrium or their carrying capacity for interest organizations far more quickly (Gray and Lowery 1996). Thus, though the stability term of the model remains of theoretical interest, it has not had empirical import in models of interest communities in stable Western democracies.

In sum, the ESA model of interest system density emphasizes contextual factors such that the number of potential constituents sets in a density-dependent manner the basic carrying capacity of political systems for organized interests. This density-dependent response function may be lowered or raised depending on the size of the political agenda of concern to different types of interests and the level of uncertainty associated with different configurations of party competition. But overall, interest populations are self-limiting as crowding suppresses birthrates and enhances death rates within guilds of organized interests.

Another implication of the model that will become important as we examine the density of health interests arises from its assumption that the density-dependent response functions of different subcommunities (also known as guilds such as health, manufacturing, and law) vary and the observation that the content of policy agendas changes over time. That is, given differences in the heterogeneity of issues within interest guilds and variations in average capacities across guilds to organize, the extent of density dependence will vary across guilds. In contrast to the conventional interpretation of the business bias in interest communities (Schattschneider 1960; Schlozman and Tierney 1986), then, the diversity of interest organizations in a community is complexly related to the distribution of interests in society and may change markedly with the size of political jurisdictions (Lowery and Gray 2004a; Lowery, Gray, and Fellowes 2005).

The Density of Health Interest Organization Communities

The first trait that is used to describe interest communities is their density or how crowded they are. The first step in measuring this trait is counting how many organizations are lobbying, which we do by counting how many health organizations in each state are registered to lobby the state legislature. This raw count of organizations does not adequately address the fact that density is a relational concept. An audience of one hundred will likely make for a crowded concert at the local pub, but that same audience will seem sparse for a concert at the football arena.

To address the relational aspect of the density, we use an indicator that measures the relationship between interest organizations and governance and is simply the number of interest organizations relative to the institutions they lobby. In the literature, the institutions of government are treated as a single entity, so the measure is simply the raw count of interest organizations divided by one state government. This measure allows for valid comparisons of the density between different interest communities and among interest communities over time.

To examine the density of health care interest organizations in the US states, we use a data set that is an extension of Gray and Lowery's list of organizations registered to lobby in the fifty states in the 1990s.[3] Lobby registration lists were gathered by mail or Web page from state agencies responsible for their maintenance. After purging the lists of state agencies in states requiring their registration, organizations registered to lobby—rather than individual lobbyists—were coded by interest content (twenty-six guilds of substantive interests) using directories of organizations and associations and the web pages of individual organizations. A second coder—the senior author—then examined the coding assignments with discrepancies resolved via discussion between the two coders.[4] The organizations in the broad health category among the complete population of guilds were then recoded by finer substantive interest using the eighteen subcategories reported in appendix 2.1 and by Lowery and Gray (2007). Following Lowery and Gray (2007) and some preliminary analyses of how these guilds tend to be arrayed for and against the several types of state health care policy initiatives we examine in later chapters, we settled on a more aggregated set of six health interests for presentation purposes: direct providers of patient care, drugs and health products, health finance, local government health agencies, health care advocacy, and health professional associations and health education institutions. Examples of each are provided in appendix 2.1.

We first examine the density of the health interest organization communities in each of the states over time. These data are summarized in figure 2.1, which shows the total number of health interest organizations in the states in 1990, 1997, 1998, and 1999. The first point to notice is the significant increase in the density of health interest organizations between 1990 and 1997, from 3,000 at the beginning of the decade to about 4,800 seven years later. In other words, more health interest organizations were registered relative to the state government in 1999 than 1990.

Figure 2.1 State Health Interest Group Density, 1990-99

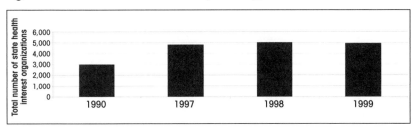

Source: Calculated by the authors.

Next, in figure 2.2, we examine the variation in the density of health interest organizations among the states in 1999, toward the end of our study period. The map shows that the number of health interest organizations ranged from a low of nine in Wyoming to a high of more than three hundred in Florida. The analyses that follow in chapters 3 through 5 sometimes utilize this simple, total number of health care interest organizations to explain variance among the states in progress toward health reforms where such organizations tend to be allied and working against other, non–health interest organizations. This measure provides the simplest form of density to interpret when used for explanatory purposes in our models of health reforms, and the raw numbers can be easily, and understandably, converted into proportions, as we show in the next section on the diversity of communities of health interest organizations.

Diversity

Density is not the only trait of populations that interests us. We are also interested in the balance of different types of interest organizations or the diversity of interest communities. If, for example, pharmaceutical interests are thought to be too well represented in state capitals, that influence might in part be mitigated with better representation by organizations representing the uninsured (Berry 1999).

The definition of diversity provided by the population ecology approach is quite straightforward. The diversity of the interest community at any one point in time is defined simply as a weighted summation of the densities of different subsets or guilds of interest organizations found in any one place or time. But once we move beyond this definition, things become more complex. This complexity arises from a unique feature of the population ecology model of density—its attention not just to individual interest organizations

Figure 2.2 Health Interest Organization Density Map, 1999

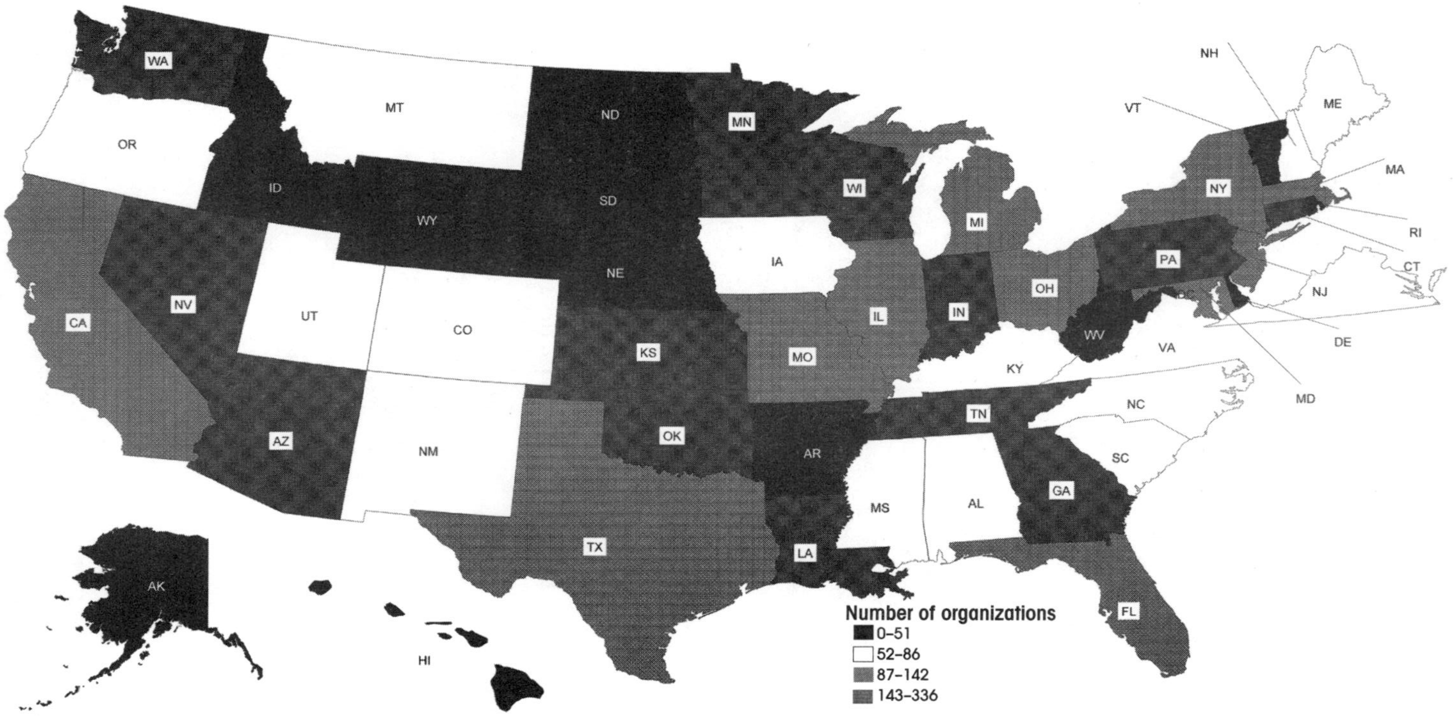

Number of organizations

- 0–51
- 52–86
- 87–142
- 143–336

but also to the number of similar organizations that are already in the interest community. Some types of organizations are more sensitive to changes in number of constituents and political and policy energy than others. Another way of saying this is that different subsets of the population of health interests have different economies of scale of representation. Indeed, Lowery, Gray, and Fellowes (2005) find that these differences in their economies of scale of representation are closely related to and reflect their differences in economies of scale of production. This means, for example, that the number of electric utility firms grows more slowly than does the number of restaurants in responses to increasing population. These differences are reflected in the number of interest organizations representing utilities and restaurants in more and less populated states.

Thus, the populations of some types of organized interests are more density dependent than others. In this interpretation, then, the diversity of the interest community is cross-sectionally a weighted summation of the densities of different subsets of lobby organizations found in a place or time. But over time that level of diversity changes in complex ways as the interest community becomes more crowded and the several guilds of organized interests respond differently to both the increased availability of resources needed for survival and the enhanced levels of competition for them (Lowery, Gray, and Fellowes 2005).

To examine the diversity of health interest organizations in the states, we start with the density of lobby registrations in our data by health organizations representing (1) direct providers of patient care, (2) manufacturers of drugs and health products, (3) health finance firms, (4) local government health agencies, (5) health care advocacy groups, and (6) health professional associations and health education institutions. These six categories, described in appendix 2.1, were aggregated upward from an even finer eighteen-category coding of the substantive interests of health organization lobby registrations.

The six categories of health interest organizations are not similar in size (Gray et al. 2005b). As seen in the first two columns of table 2.2, 50 percent of the health registrations by organizations in the average state in 1997 were concerned with direct providers of patient care, a proportion that fell only slightly to 49 percent in 1999. The next largest category of registrations contained drug and health product organizations, followed by health professional associations and health education institutions, health care advocacy groups, health finance organizations, and local government health groups and agencies, which made up only 3 percent of the health interest community in the average state in 1997 and 3 percent in 1999. There are other types of health interest organizations, but these six categories constitute the major categories.

Table 2.2 Subguild Means (percent)

Subguild Type	State Mean, 1997	State Mean, 1999
Direct patient care providers	50.14	48.80
Drugs and health products	18.22	18.24
Health finance	7.32	7.43
Local government health	2.83	2.67
Health care advocacy	9.03	10.31
Health professional associations and education	12.46	12.55

Source: Calculated by the authors.

Next, it is important to establish that these six subguilds are distinct populations and not just six categories of a single population that grow and shrink together. Some evidence on this issue is reported in the correlation matrices of densities of the six subguilds in the fifty states in 1997 and 1999, which are presented in table 2.3. These correlations are positive and large, but not so large as to conclude that the six subguilds grow or decline together as part of a larger population (Gray et al. 2005b). As seen in the density data by subguild presented in appendix 2.2, big states like New York or California are going to have many more lobby registrations by health organizations of all six types than will a small state like Vermont.

We show, in the remaining chapters, that each of our models of health reform policies arrays different guilds and subguilds of interest organizations based upon their position for or against the policy. It is this balance between the population of advocates and opponents that should determine the ability of interest organizations to influence policy change or maintain the status quo.

Communities of Contributors: The Connection between Organized Interests and Political Action Committees

Although the theoretical and empirical focus of this book centers on the community of health organizations registered to lobby their state legislatures, it is important to remember that lobbying is not the only way for health organizations to participate in the process of advocating for or against health reform. There also exists a community of health organizations, as well as business and other groups, in each state making contributions to candidates during the electoral process. Perhaps surprisingly, the political science literature provides a rather mixed picture of the relationship between the lobbying activities of organized interests and the campaign finance activities of political action committees (PACs). It is often assumed that campaign donations are

Table 2.3 Subguild Intercorrelations

1997	Direct Patient Care Providers	Drugs and Health Products	Health Finance	Local Government Health	Health Care Advocacy
Drugs and health products	0.82				
Health finance	0.82	0.75			
Local government health	0.62	0.56	0.45		
Health care advocacy	0.78	0.79	0.69	0.62	
Health professional and education	0.84	0.81	0.77	0.56	0.83
1999	Direct Patient Care Providers	Drugs and Health Products	Health Finance	Local Government Health	Health Care Advocacy
Drugs and health products	0.85				
Health finance	0.80	0.71			
Local government health	0.75	0.73	0.56		
Health care advocacy	0.80	0.76	0.57	0.77	
Health professional and education	0.85	0.86	0.72	0.74	0.83

Source: Calculated by the authors.

an integral lobbying strategy of organized interests. PACs, some argue, may purchase policy or at least the access needed to influence the elected officials making policy. Still, scholarly research more often than not fails to find a tight connection between the two influence activities (Berry 1977; Wright 1985; Schlozman and Tierney 1986; Gais and Walker 1991; Nownes and Freeman 1998).

The bulk of the extant literature on PACs and lobbying suggests that explanations of PAC formation and the density of lobbying communities are not as straightforward as we might expect. Despite findings that PAC contributions can influence votes under very specific circumstances (Quinn and Shapiro 1991; Godwin 1988; Wilhite and Theilmann 1987), or on minor issues (Grenzke 1989), or on narrow, technical issues (Frendreis and Waterman 1985), the most thorough study found that PAC contributions had little impact on legislative voting (Wright 2004). These studies have led many scholars to believe that PAC donations are more about access than about purchasing policy (Lowery and Brasher 2004). Still, even this reinterpretation of the role of PACs in the policy process is faced with a significant conundrum. That is, many organizations that lobby do not contribute to electoral campaigns, and many organizations that contribute to campaigns do not lobby. Indeed, surveys of organized interests lobbying in Washington found little connection between lobbying and contributing to campaigns (Berry 1977; Wright 1985; Schlozman and Tierney 1986; Gais and Walker 1991). Survey research at the state level found similar results; less than half of lobbying organizations contributed to campaigns (Nownes and Freeman 1998). If the two types of influence organizations represent different populations, then it is hard to maintain the access hypothesis. Instead, these studies seem to indicate that lobbying and contributing to campaigns are relatively independent strategies of influence.

More recently, however, several studies (Tripathi, Ansolabehere, and Snyder 2002; Gray and Lowery 1997; Lowery et al. 2009) highlight evidence pointing to a much stronger relationship between lobbying by organized interests and the campaign activities of PACs.[5] It now seems that competition for lobbying access drives PAC formation and levels of campaign contributions at both the national and state levels.

First, Tripathi, Ansolabehere, and Snyder (2002) analyzed the convergence of organizations registered to lobby Congress and executive agencies in 1997–98 and organizations donating to House of Representative campaigns through PACs during 1997–98. In terms of interest organization numbers, their findings support the weak link between lobbying and PAC donations. They found that 74.5 percent of all organizations registered to lobby had no PAC, and 52.8 percent of PACs were not affiliated with a registered lobbying organization. Instead of stopping there, however, they looked beyond numbers of organizations to the amount of money they contributed. Here they found that 85.7 percent of all campaign contributions were donated by PACs that were affiliated with organizations also registered to lobby. So if we base our analysis on the size of the contributions, PAC donations can still be viewed as one of several lobbying tactics in which an organization engages.

Second, a 1997 study by Gray and Lowery further exploring the assumption that PAC contributions are a lobbying tactic found that PAC contributions are especially crucial in crowded organized interest environments, where it is more difficult to gain access to elected officials. By examining their hypothesis at the state level, Gray and Lowery observed variation that could not be seen at the national level (only one interest system) or over time (little variation in total number of national PACs over time). They examined their hypothesis in two ways. First, using surveys of organized interest leaders, they found that those who viewed their lobbying community as crowded and competitive were more likely to be affiliated with a PAC. Next, using aggregate numbers of organizations registered to lobby and numbers of PACs, they found a significant, positive, convex relationship between the number of PACs and the number of lobby registrations by organizations. So, as the density of lobbying organizations increases, the population of PACs in a given community increases.

Third, Lowery and colleagues (2009) expanded on these studies to understand the relationship between PAC contributions and lobbying on health care policies. Using data collected from the National Institute on Money in State Politics and described in detail in appendix 2.3, they focused specifically on the health policy arena to address several questions arising from Tripathi, Ansolabehere, and Snyder (2002) and Gray and Lowery (1997). First, they were able to replicate the Tripathi and colleagues finding at the state level. The relationship between national PAC activity and lobbying in all policy domains was mirrored with state health PAC contributions and lobby registrations by health organizations, as seen in figures 2.3 and 2.4. In terms of simple numbers of organizations, these results were somewhat similar to Tripathi and colleagues' findings. Only 14 percent of the 10,755 active health interest organizations have both a PAC and a lobbying organization. Tripathi and colleagues found that 20 percent of national-level organizations have both a lobbyist and a PAC (2002, 133). Thus, the conventional wisdom of a lobby organization armed with its mighty PAC occurs only one-fifth of the time at the national level. For state-level health organizations, the number falls to only 14 percent. In contrast, unaffiliated or free-standing PACs at the state level account for 45 percent of such organizations, and organizations registered to lobby but lacking a PAC account for another 41 percent. Here, the state results depart from those at the national level. Tripathi and colleagues found that lobby-only organizations predominated, occurring 58 percent of the time. PAC-only organizations made up only 22 percent of all organizations at the national level.

The picture changes markedly, however, when we look at the actual political activity of state health PACs. It is the many fewer affiliated PACs (those connected to a health interest organization) that provide the lion's share of funds to state candidates. Although connected or affiliated PACs accounted for only 23.8 percent of all health PACs, they contributed more than $34 million, or 76 percent of all contributions. In contrast, though unaffiliated PACs accounted for 76.1 percent of the PAC population in health, they made only $11 million in contributions, or 24 percent of all state contributions.[6] These

Figure 2.3 Numbers of Health PACs and Interest Organizations in the States, 1998

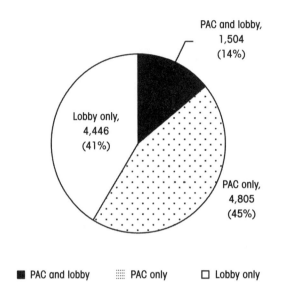

PAC and lobby,
1,504
(14%)

Lobby only,
4,446
(41%)

PAC only,
4,805
(45%)

■ PAC and lobby   ⬚ PAC only   □ Lobby only

Source: Calculated by the authors using data from the National Institute on Money in State Politics.

aggregate numbers are reflected in the differences between mean contribution levels of nonconnected and connected health PACs. The mean contribution for nonconnected PACs was only $2,319, whereas the mean contribution for connected PACs was nearly ten times larger ($23,067). In terms of both total volume and average size, the state contribution activity of connected PACs dwarfs that of nonconnected PACs in health. In terms of PAC activity, the state health results parallel those at the national level, where affiliated PACs contributed even more disproportionately, giving 86 percent of the total PAC contributions in all sectors (Tripathi, Ansolabehere, and Snyder 2002, 133). PAC activity is largely the province of organizations already engaged in lobbying. Given this connection, it seems reasonable to interpret such activity as a strategy designed to reinforce lobbying or as an adjunct of lobbying.

Lowery and colleagues (2009) also found support for Gray and Lowery's 1997 finding of a positive, convex relationship between the numbers of PACs and lobbying registrations, or that lobby registrations primarily drive PAC

Figure 2.4 Contributions of Health PACs and Interest Organizations in the States, 1998

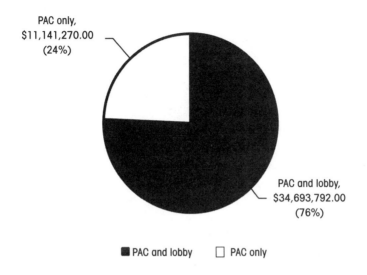

PAC only,
$11,141,270.00
(24%)

PAC and lobby,
$34,693,792.00
(76%)

■ PAC and lobby   □ PAC only

Source: Calculated by the authors using data from the National Institute on Money in State Politics.

density and contributions. Finally, they found that competition in specific policy arenas (or local competition) rather than overall interest system competition is what drives the relationship between lobbying registrations and PACs. They concluded with the notion that PAC densities depend upon lobbying registrations and little else, positing that "the dynamics of the PAC system are a secondary effect of the process governing lobbying, as described by Gray and Lowery's (1996) ESA model" (Lowery et al. 2009, 19).

Conclusions

Chapter 2 provided an introduction to the ESA model that guides our exploration of the effects of interest organizations in the health care reform process. This model—the now-dominant model in the literature used to understand the density and diversity of interest communities—underlies much of our consideration of the policy influence of different subsets of interest organizations in the remaining chapters. Still, these chapters are more about policy influence than about how interest populations form.

However, there is a strong connection between the ESA model and the models of policy influence we develop in later chapters. That is, one of the core assumptions of the ESA model is that political and policy uncertainty—the energy, or demand, term of the ESA model—draw interest organizations to the policy process, an assumption that has received considerable empirical support during the last fifteen years. Thus, the model assumes that interest organizations react more to the policy agenda than create it in the first place. What they then do when they react to policy initiatives placed on the policy agenda by politicians is the focus of the bulk of our analysis, especially so the balance or diversity of different types of interests that are drawn into the policy process. Of particular importance, however, these influence models are predicated on the ESA assumption that health interests are largely reactive to exogenously generated policy proposals.

More prosaically, if nevertheless important, this chapter has also introduced our data on the structure of health interest communities in the fifty states, including the density and diversity of health-related interests that are used in the remaining chapters to develop and test models of the influence of organized interests on health policy. Our review of the population data in this chapter has highlighted significant variations in this structure across both time and space. These variations, both in the rapid increase in health interest organizations over time and in the differences between states in terms of the size and composition of the health interest organization community, are what will allow us to test our models of health reform in chapters 3 through 5.

Notes

1. Olson's analysis is incorrect in that interest organizations do die, sometimes at alarming rates that reach as high as 50 percent over a decade (Gray and Lowery 1995a; also see Nownes and Lapinski 2005).

2. Olson's model has attracted plenty of criticism at the individual level over the years. Scholars have shown that organizations with members are quite adept at overcoming barriers to collective action (see Salisbury 1969; Walker 1991; Rosenstone and Hansen 1993). Research has also shown that citizens have a range of membership incentives—and varied interpretations of those incentives—that both mitigate free riding and the by-product consequences of the use of narrowly material selective incentives (see Moe 1980; Hansen 1985).

3. Fortunately, previous work indicates that the stringency of state lobbying registration requirements has little impact on the density (Lowery and Gray 1994, 1997) and diversity (Gray and Lowery 1998b) of state interest communities.

4. Only 1.58 percent of the 35,928 organizational lobby registrations in 1997 could not be coded by substantive interest.

5. Note that our study and the literature cited were carried out before the advent of the super-PACs at either the state or national level.

6. This three-to-one ratio of contribution dollars from connected PACs to dollars from unconnected PACs is also true for each party. Connected PACs account for 74 percent of contributions to Democrats in the states and 77 percent of contributions to Republicans. Contributions to Republicans ($25,368,300) somewhat exceed those to Democrats ($20,222,100). Note that these numbers exclude smaller contributions to third parties. There are no significant differences in the two-party distribution of PAC contributions between nonconnected and connected PACs.

CHAPTER 3

State Pharmacy Assistance Programs as Innovations

At the end of 2003 President George W. Bush and the Republican Congress passed the Medicare Prescription Drug, Improvement, and Modernization Act (MMA), the largest increase in social spending since the Great Society, which was estimated to cost at least $400 billion over ten years. The law began as an effort to add prescription drug coverage to Medicare, a problem that had been recognized for the previous thirty-eight years, and an issue highlighted by President Bill Clinton in his State of the Union Address in 1999. The Clinton administration and Democrats in Congress, blessed with a budgetary surplus, had attempted to add drug coverage in the 1990s but were thwarted by congressional Republicans. Drug coverage for seniors then became a campaign issue in the 2000 election, with Bush and Democratic candidate Al Gore each proposing competing plans. During President Bush's first two years in office, the Democrats managed to fight off his attempts at Medicare "modernization," which involved privatization as well as drug coverage. But after Republicans gained full control in November 2002, his administration's plans for Medicare faced a friendlier Congress, as well as a mounting budget deficit.

The fight over MMA mobilized more than five hundred interest groups (Heaney 2006), many of which spent lavishly on lobbying and were rewarded by generous treatment in the bill.[1] The pharmaceutical industry, represented by the Pharmaceutical Research and Manufacturers of America, spent big and won big: no competitive bidding on drug prices, a ban on drug importation from Canada, and a sizable new subsidized market of seniors. The pharmaceutical industry helpfully bankrolled issue ads on the MMA proposal for the Republicans in the 2002 elections, giving them a three-to-one advantage on issue ad spending (Morgan and Campbell 2011b, 131). The managed care industry and private insurers also emerged victorious as the Republicans' version of "modernization" meant private-sector management of the drug benefit, $14 billion in enticements that would go to those private vendors offering health plans (labeled Medicare Advantage plans) for the Medicare market (Oliver, Lee, and Lipton 2004), and a demonstration plan for them to compete with traditional Medicare for customers. The insurance industry sank millions into lobbying and campaign contributions. Employers won because they got $70 billion in subsidies to not drop retiree drug coverage they were already offering (Oberlander 2007). Providers—physicians and hospitals—got improved reimbursement rates, including $21 billion for providers in rural areas (Oliver, Lee, and Lipton 2004), while conservative business groups achieved the authorization of medical savings accounts. At the last minute AARP endorsed the bill as "too good an opportunity to pass up" (Oberlander 2007, 192) and in return won concessions that made the bill more palatable to it. As Heaney (2006, 929) put it, "When the weight of public sentiment called for a prescription drug benefit under Medicare, the benefit was purchased at the expense of a wide array of pork-barrel benefits for doctors, rural health providers, insurance companies, pharmaceutical manufacturers, and others." His sentiments about the MMA being a triumph of private interests is echoed by Oberlander (2007) and Morgan and Campbell (2011b). Hall and Houweling's (2006, 34) judgment about the impact of private interests on the bill is more nuanced, but even they noted that "one cannot conclude that campaign money bought the healthcare industry the legislation it wanted, but money did receive robust representation."

The winners overrode other reputably influential organized interests— longtime Democratic champions who could not tolerate the "privatizing" of Medicare elements in the bill and antitax conservatives who were upset that their party had created a huge new entitlement whose price tag ballooned overnight. Worse yet, the Republicans identified no financing source at all for the large additional cost, even though the budgetary surplus had already vanished (Starr 2011, 149). Surely each of these interests would have preferred very different kinds of legislation to address the high costs of prescription drugs, with the liberal Democrats preferring across-the-board coverage for all Medicare recipients. Senator Ted Kennedy declared on the floor of the Senate that the MMA was "a right-wing Republican assault on Medicare in the guise of a prescription drug program, . . . a fat deal for HMOs [health maintenance organizations] and pharmaceutical companies—and a raw deal for the elderly" (cited by Morgan and Campbell 2011b, 140). Even the senior beneficiaries were not such clear winners as their drug benefit had a "doughnut hole" in the middle that could not be bridged by another insurance plan.[2] Additionally, "modernization" of Medicare introduced means testing of beneficiaries for the first time.[3] In a poll taken the week the bill was signed into law, 47 percent of seniors opposed the changes to Medicare, and only 26 percent approved (Oliver, Lee, and Lipton 2004).

An Overview of State Pharmacy Assistance Programs

Given the length of time it took for a prescription drug benefit to be added to Medicare and the consensus interpretation of the MMA's politics as a triumph of the health care and pharmaceutical industries and other conservative interests over public opinion and longtime Democratic supporters of such a benefit, it may surprise some to know that by 2004 fully thirty-four of the fifty states had already established programs providing prescription drug assistance to low-income seniors.[4] Such programs were targeted at the near-poor elderly (and sometimes the disabled, depending on the state) whose incomes were too high to qualify for Medicaid. Maine and New Jersey were the first to provide drug coverage for their seniors in 1975. Maryland, Pennsylvania, Rhode Island, and Illinois joined them during the next decade. Five more states enacted drug legislation by the end of the 1980s—Connecticut, New York, Michigan, Wyoming, and Vermont. Interest at this point may have been related to events leading up to the passage of the Catastrophic Coverage Act of 1988, which included a plan to phase in prescription drug coverage for Medicare beneficiaries. The 1988 act itself was judged a catastrophe and was repealed by Congress rather quickly. The drug assistance movement was then quiescent in the states until 1996. But then it took off again, with twenty states adopting prescription drug policies between 1996 and 2004. Nearly 1.7 million were served by these programs in 2003 (NCSL 2004); nearly three-quarters of the recipients were located in just five states—New York, Pennsylvania, New Jersey, Illinois, and Massachusetts. A study sponsored by the Commonwealth Fund estimated that state pharmaceutical assistance programs (SPAPs) provided prescription drug coverage to approximately 16 percent of potentially eligible persons in their states in 2002 (Trail et al. 2004). But this average varied widely, from more than 40 percent in Pennsylvania and a few other states to fewer than 10 percent in states with more recently established SPAPs. And adopting these policies was not a one-time event on the states' part. Between 1996 and 2004, sixteen states enacted laws expanding their original pharmacy assistance programs, usually making them more generous. Between 2000 and 2004, three states adopted legislation expanding their programs a second time.

Even after passage of the MMA in 2003, leaders of both parties in the states with the most generous pharmacy assistance programs pledged to maintain them. Two weeks before the Medicare drug bill was signed by President Bush, Pennsylvania's governor Ed Rendell signed a bill supported by both political parties that increased enrollment in the state's program from 234,000 to 340,000. A Republican leader in the Illinois Senate complained that "instead of emphasizing the good work being done by states and encouraging states to continue, the federal government came up with a one-size-fits-all Potomac solution" (quoted by Hernandez and Pear 2004). Thus, policymakers in states shouldering the largest burden of expense for their seniors' drug bills did not seem to expect that their states' programs would cease once Part D was implemented.

The federal battle over prescription drugs was joined again in 2009–10, when President Obama and the Democratic Congress attempted to close the doughnut hole for seniors as an element of the Patient Protection and Affordable Care Act (ACA). As part of his "co-opt the opposition" strategy, the president got AARP on board early with a promise that any reform bill would eliminate Medicare's gap in coverage of prescription drugs (Calmes 2009). More newsworthy was the fact that the president made an $80 billion agreement (over ten years) with the pharmaceutical industry on behalf of his administration and the Senate Finance Committee whereby the industry agreed to a series of pledges, including a 50 percent price discount on drugs purchased by Medicare beneficiaries in the doughnut hole. The deal reduced the amount of federal subsidy required to close the hole entirely by 2020 and expands the pool of seniors who will be buying drugs from the industry in the future. In return, the Obama administration opposed drug importation and further rebates on drugs for Medicare beneficiaries and agreed to provisions the industry demanded on regulation of so-called biologics.

With these agreements in place, the pharmaceutical industry threw its very substantial weight behind the ACA; in return, the industry should gain 32 million new customers who will buy drugs from them. The pharmaceutical industry spent an estimated $100 million on TV advertising, grassroots organizing, and other marketing efforts in support of Obama's health reform (Abelson 2010), whereas in 1993–94 their money was spent against Clinton's version of health reform. No one ad better symbolizes the difference between the Clinton years and the Obama years than the $4 million reunion of Harry and Louise around the kitchen table, paid for in 2009–10 by the Pharmaceutical Research and Manufacturers of America and Families USA. This time, Harry and Louise were speaking positively about health care reform; the previous poster couple for opposition to government health care now thought "it was about time" that "we get good coverage people can afford, coverage they can get even if they have a preexisting condition" (quoted by Serafini 2009a, 28).

Since Part D of MMA went into effect in 2006, most states have reacted by converting their existing SPAPs into "wraparound coverage," which most often pays for the enrollee's monthly premium, coinsurance expenses, and annual deductible. The federal program allows states to save money by substituting federal Medicare dollars for state SPAP dollars for low-income beneficiaries, netting about $600 million per year (NCSL 2009, app. 1). Four states—Arizona, Florida, Michigan, and Minnesota—responded by shutting down their SPAPs entirely and letting their near-needy seniors rely solely on Medicare's Part D (NCSL 2010c). Seven states have added new SPAPs since the enactment of MMA, some at the same time as they began a Medicare wraparound program. Thus, state activity continued in this area even after Medicare's Part D had supposedly taken care of seniors' prescription cost problems.

However, future state action will not be as autonomous as in the period we examine in this chapter (1990–2001), because "clawback" provisions of the MMA demand money from the states and heavily influence what they can do in their own programs (see Weissert and Miller 2005; Weissert and Weissert 2006). Moreover, a recent study of enrollment shortfall in Medicare Part D (Davidoff et al. 2010) warns that closing the doughnut hole may have the perverse impact of reducing enrollment among nonsubsidized beneficiaries due to higher premiums and among low-income subsidized beneficiaries due to barriers to enrollment. Thus, behavioral strategies in addition to the monetary ones incorporated into ACA and SPAPs may be needed to ensure that all seniors reap the benefits accorded by the ACA.

So why did thirty-four states, already spending heavily on other health care programs like Medicaid and the Children's Health Insurance Program (CHIP), decide to offer pharmacy benefits to low-income seniors?[5] It is not as if needy seniors are a mobile group about to exit for another state if not served; nor is this a benefit designed to attract new residents with skills needed in the workforce. Further, the health of seniors has traditionally been a federal responsibility under Medicare via its link to the Social Security program. Quite clearly, it was Medicare's failure to cover prescription drugs in the first place that created the demand for the states to assist elderly citizens. But this simple fact begs the underlying question posed by the conventional explanation of health care reform as being taken over by special interests. Why were the same special interests that were so effective in delaying meaningful prescription drug coverage at the national level for so long and then shaping its final passage so as to disproportionately benefit themselves so incapable of stopping the majority of states from passing somewhat similar legislation in a straightforward way?

To be sure, not all states adopted prescription drug programs. And among those offering financial help, seven states delayed implementation, capped enrollment, or suspended new enrollment due to budgetary problems between 2001 (when our study ended) and 2010. And as noted, four states quit operating SPAPs entirely after the MMA was implemented. But when compared with efforts of the federal government during the last thirty-five years, the states' continuing efforts to assist seniors with the costs of prescription drugs are impressive. Their programs have not been turned upside down by organized interests so that they help the interests more than the needy seniors; that is, they have not been captured. Moreover, the variation from one state to another allows us to test a number of hypotheses about the determinants of state health policy in the pharmacy area. We discuss measures of the SPAPs in the next section, followed by an examination of a set of hypotheses and the theories that guide them. Heckman models are then employed to test the hypotheses with data on the adoption, revision, and generosity of SPAPs from 1990 through 2001. We find little evidence that organized interests had direct influence on the adoption of SPAPs, but we provide evidence that such interests did influence their revision and generosity. We examine these findings in light of the balance of democratic and nondemocratic influences on state health care policy.

Measures of Policy Activity on State Pharmaceutical Assistance Programs

It is unlikely that the full period running from the earliest adoptions in 1975 by New Jersey and Maine through Iowa's 2009 passage of the program is equally compelling, given our focus on organized interests. As figure 3.1 shows, eleven of the thirty-four states providing drug assistance established their programs before 1990. Thus, their legislation predates both the rapid growth of prescription drug costs during the 1990s and the rush of organized interests into the business of health care lobbying associated with the introduction and subsequent defeat of the Clinton health care plan. Moreover, there is a gap from the 1989 legislation and the next in Massachusetts in 1996. There are also good reasons to think that the more recent adoptions are somewhat unusual. That is, after the peak year of adoption of 2001, when six states adopted, annual adoptions declined, and by 2002 pharmacy assistance

Figure 3.1 New and Cumulative Number of State Pharmaceutical Assistance Programs, 1974–2009

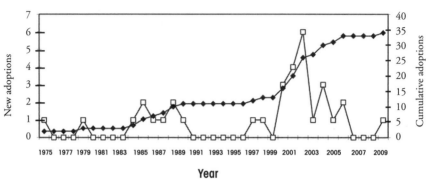

Year

Source: Calculated by the authors.

programs became enmeshed in the politics of state budget crises. Beginning in 2003 and continuing into the present, state activity on pharmacy assistance has been directed toward Medicare wraparound programs, which takes us into a whole different era of federal–state programs. Moreover, we are determined to study only state-initiated, state-funded programs in this book, because their politics is fundamentally different from those programs in which the federal government is involved (see Barrilleaux and Brace 2007). For these reasons, as well as because of data limitations earlier and later in the time series, we focus on new adoptions, program changes, and the generosity of state pharmaceutical assistance programs from 1990 to 2001.[6] This period should provide us the cleanest test of the influence of organized interests.[7]

Measures of the Dependent Variables

We are interested in three traits of state pharmacy assistance programs as our dependent variables. A full list of sources for all the measures is provided in appendix 3.1.

Measure 1. The first is simple adoption and maintenance of a prescription drug program. More specifically, we stipulate the adoption of the program among the first eleven states and focus on the twenty new adoptions occurring from 1990 through 2001. This measure uses a simple dichotomous variable coded 1 to indicate that a state maintained a program in each of the respective years examined.

Measure 2. Second, we examine revisions in ongoing state programs. As noted above, many states did not stand pat on their initial legislation even in the face of recent federal activity on prescription drugs. Indeed, sixteen states have enacted new laws expanding their original pharmacy assistance programs since 1996. And since 2000, three states have adopted new legislation altering their programs in major ways a second time. We measure program revisions between 1990 and 2001 with a dichotomous variable indicating that a state's program in a given year is a revision of its original form.[8]

Measure 3. Third and especially important, we examine the programmatic generosity of SPAPs from 1990 through 2001, including the generosity of programs adopted before 1990. That is, even without major program revisions, states continually tinker with their prescription drug programs, sometimes making them more generous and other times less so. We measure generosity with an annual item index of standardized scores on three traits of state drug programs. The first is the *extent of coverage.* Programs vary across states and over time, with many covering only seniors more than sixty-two years of age (coded 1), others covering seniors and the disabled (coded 2), and those imposing no age or physical limit to coverage (coded 3). The second trait concerns *income limits.* That is, states limit program eligibility to singles or families who are needy, but not so needy as to be on Medicaid, using the federal poverty line (FPL) as the criterion for cutoff. In 2001, for example, the cap on eligibility ranged from 90 percent of the FPL in Arkansas to 500 percent in Massachusetts, with the latter being far more generous. Our indicator of income limit, then, is the FPL limit of a program by state-year. Third, states impose a number of *cost-sharing requirements* on recipients, which may deter enrollment. Requiring a payment up front—a premium, an enrollment fee, or a deductible—has been found to have the greatest negative impact on enrollment (Crystal et al. 2003, 12). Such requirements were assigned the code of 1. Coinsurance charges (i.e., a percentage of the drug's cost), limiting the kinds of drugs that are subsidized or the number of prescriptions filled per month, were coded as 2 because these rules are deemed slightly less onerous. Requiring modest flat copays for each prescription was coded 3 because this requirement would have the least financial impact on recipients. And last, programs with no limits were assigned a code of 4. Again, the higher score indicates programs with requirements designed to attract low-income people, not turn them away. These standardized items were combined in an index of generosity, with higher scores indicating greater generosity.

Innovation and ESA Theories Contribute Concepts to Explain SPAPs' Adoption

The major contribution of this chapter lies in the case we examine, state pharmacy assistance programs whose politics have not previously been examined, and our measures of the density and diversity of interest communities derived from Energy Stability Area (ESA) theory. Moreover, the additional hypotheses we test are part of a long tradition of innovation research. For our purpose, state pharmacy assistance programs are the innovation, beginning in 1975 with two states and spreading eventually to thirty-four by 2009. But in an effort to study the *content* of the policy that is diffusing across the states, we also examine major program revisions as well as the programmatic generosity of the SPAPs. Many of these hypotheses will be the same as those for the initial innovation, but prior theory tells us that enacting a new law is a more salient event than amending an existing law or modifying details of programmatic limits. And we know that organized interests have more influence where the salience of the policy activity is low than where salience is high (Lowery and Brasher 2004, 172–73). Behind closed doors anything can happen between producer and provider groups and beneficiary groups—they may all come together to advocate for broader enrollment designs or the earlier enemies may tighten enrollment greatly. And in the revision process, the comment "the devil is in the details" fits well. Health industry groups have an advantage over outside advocacy and patient groups because they do know the details very well.

In predicting policy adoptions, we expect that the internal determinants model of innovation holds the most promise in this case. Specifically, we examine measures of the intensity of the policy problem in the states, their capacity to address the problem, the public's preferences for state action, and partisan and ideological influences, as discussed in chapter 1. External determinants seem less plausible in the case of SPAPs than with policies we examine in the next chapter. There was no federal incentive to innovate during our study period and no plausible interstate competition over seniors. External diffusion measures were developed for emulation of one's neighbors who had SPAPs as well as for national policy developments that may have heightened the salience of the policy. The latter is a type of top-down vertical diffusion.

VARIABLES, SET ONE: ORGANIZED INTEREST GROUPS

Among the internal determinants, we are particularly interested in the role of organized interests. The literature provides competing assessments of the impact of the density and diversity of interest communities on public policy (Lowery and Brasher 2004). To some, the presence of large numbers of business interests is sufficient evidence that business must exercise undue influence (Schattschneider 1960; Schlozman and Tierney 1986). But other scholars argue that excessive presence within an interest system represents weakness rather than strength. That is, some core interest must be threatened before they willingly incur the costs of lobbying (Heinz et al. 1993). Still others suggest that whether the density and diversity of an interest system indicates policy dominance or weakness depends on both the unity of the interest community and the unity and direction of public opinion (Smith 2000).

Indeed, the literature on state public policy offers confirmatory findings on the influence of organized interests in the area of health policy most closely associated with SPAPs, that of Medicaid. Grogan (1994) found that interest pressure affected state Medicaid policy decisions. As she predicted, the strength of provider interest groups had the greatest impact on benefit coverage decisions, a moderate impact for categorical eligibility, and limited impact on financial eligibility decisions. Barrilleaux and Miller (1988) reported that the diversity of the interest system was positively associated with Medicaid effort, defined as the proportion of total state personal income spent on Medicaid vendor payments (minus the federal share of Medicaid payments). Perhaps most relevant is Pracht and Moore's (2003, 31) analysis of organized interests and pharmacy reimbursement rates in state Medicaid programs, which found that the participation rate of pharmacists in state affiliates of the American Pharmaceutical Association was positively associated with Medicaid pharmacy reimbursement rates. Given these findings, it seems quite plausible to expect that the density and diversity of the health interest community in the states will influence their pharmacy assistance policies.

This set of independent variables addresses our core concerns about organized interests. We employ two sets of variables tapping the absolute and relative presence of organized interests on lobbying rolls. Both are based on state lobby registration data collected by Gray and Lowery (1996) and the health lobby data recoded by Gray and colleagues (2005b). State lobby registrations were initially coded into twenty-six guilds of substantive interests, one of which was health policy. Fully 3,904, or 13.3 percent, of all registered organizations in 1990 were coded as having some health interest, broadly defined.[9] Registrations by health organizations increased to 5,658 and 5,817 in 1997 and 1999, respectively, while their proportions of the total interest system grew to 15.8 and 15.7 percent. The health organizations were then recoded into eighteen finer categories of substantive interest.[10] The final aspect of this data set that we consider is the distinction Gray and Lowery (1996) draw between for-profit and not-for-profit interest guilds. That is, they group the twenty-six guilds of substantive interests into two larger superguilds roughly representing the profit (e.g., manufacturing and agriculture) and nonprofit (e.g., religion and local government) sectors of the economy. In all three years, roughly 75 percent of lobby registrations represented the profit sector.

The impact of group density. The first trait of interest is the absolute size or *density* of the health guild, under the expectation that simply having more organizations attentive to health care will promote (or impede) the adoption, expansion, and generosity of any health program. The mean number of health registrations in the states was 115 in 1999, ranging from 12 in Wyoming to 362 in Florida. But not all such interests may be concerned about or supportive of prescription policies for seniors.

The impact of group advocates. Thus, we also need to consider the *diversity* of health interests. Three sets of health interests may be especially concerned about drug assistance policies. The first are drug companies whose products will be subsidized by SPAPs. Pharmaceutical firms may not like the criticism they receive when prescription assistance bills are debated, but they also directly benefit as more customers can purchase drugs. Thus, they should be supportive of such programs. The second set of proponents is health advocacy groups who generally support prescription assistance programs benefiting clients, members, and the public. The third set is an array of other possible advocates.

The impact of other possible advocates. More difficult to assess are the interests of health finance organizations—health plans, health business services, employer health coalitions, and insurance companies. On balance, we think that these organizations benefit from externalizing some costs of health care from their members or customers onto the public sector. Hence, we expect they will be at least weakly supportive of SPAPs.

We measure the size of these three subguilds (pharmacy, health advocacy, and health finance) as proportions of the health sector so as to avoid collinearity arising from large states simply having more of all kinds of interests. The proportions were 15.4, 10.3, and 7.8 percent in 1999, but ranged widely across the states.

The impact of organized opponents. The third trait of the interest system we examine focuses on those who might oppose prescription programs. Perhaps the key source of *opposition* arises from those paying taxes to support such programs. The business community is typically opposed to higher taxes (Smith 2000) and therefore against redistributive programs. Accordingly, we expect business to be the major source of opposition to these programs. We measure its relative size with the proportion of lobby registrations coming from the for-profit sector. In 1999, this ranged from 59 percent in California to 83 percent in Oklahoma.

Measurement issues. Fortunately, the last indicator—the proportion of the interest community drawn from the for-profit sector—has been extremely static during the last three decades (Gray and Lowery 1996, 103). We use, then, the average of the 1990 and 1999 proportions for all years in our sample. But selecting measures for the other aspects of density and diversity is more difficult given data limitations. One route is to assume that interest communities are largely static over the period of our sample. This is not an entirely unreasonable assumption given that the 1990, 1997, and 1999 values of these variables are strongly correlated. The strength of this measure is that it builds on actual numbers of lobby registrations by organizations in the states.

Its weakness, however, is that it cannot account for some potentially important changes in the health interest community over time. On average, for example, drug interests made up only 10.3 percent of health registrations in 1990, but 17.0 percent in 1999. To account for these changes, we generated annual estimates of the size of the health guild and its proportions from the pharmacy, health advocacy, and health finance subguilds using a variant of Gray and Lowery's ESA model of interest system density described in chapter 2. This estimation procedure is described in more detail in appendix 3.2. The weakness of this measure, however, is that it is based on *estimates* from the ESA model. In a sense, these annual estimates tap the central tendency of states or their capacity to support lobby registrations of a given type, given the size of their economies and how they change over time. The estimates do not account for how political agendas cool to health issues depress lobbying while those that are more receptive promote it. Of our two possible sets of measures, then, one has limited temporal variation but is based on actual registration numbers. The other provides annual variation but is a better measure of capacity for lobbying. On balance, we believe the annual estimated measures will be more accurate, and we therefore employ them in this analysis.

The impact of AARP membership. We employ one additional measure of organized interests that is not based on the Gray-Lowery data set: the proportion of a state's senior population that belongs to AARP.[11] Seniors are most often the beneficiaries of pharmaceutical assistance programs, and thus they should strongly support them. AARP is known for being a highly effective lobby for its members and for seniors in general. It seems reasonable to expect, then, that states with higher proportions of senior membership in AARP will be more likely to adopt and maintain SPAPs.

VARIABLE SET TWO: THE PROBLEM ENVIRONMENT

A second set of hypotheses examines the objective need for state action to address the pharmaceutical cost problem for seniors. We look at three specific claims about the problem environment surrounding SPAPs.

The cost of drugs. The key pressure driving state lawmakers to help low-income seniors pay for their prescription drugs was the increase in their cost. Between 1990 and 1998 the *average annual increase* in expenditures for prescription drugs was 11.9 percent nationwide (Hovey and Hovey 2004, 262). But this varied from 15.4 percent in Nevada to 10.3 percent in California.[12] We expect that lawmakers in states with greater increases in per capita drug costs will feel more pressure from constituents to provide assistance to seniors in need.

Unfortunately, state-level data on the costs of prescription drugs were available for only four years within our twelve-year study period: 1990, 1991, 1993, and 1998. Annual values for the other years were interpolated from these data. Fortunately, the relative differences in the average costs of prescription drugs across the states seem to be quite stable over time despite the rapid increase in average national costs over time.[13] So, while we should not rely too heavily on our year-to-year measure of drug costs within any one state, it should allow us to validly distinguish states with relatively high costs from those with relatively low costs. The former should be more likely to adopt, revise, and have more generous prescription programs.

The size of the senior population. The size of a state's senior population is surely expected to be an indicator of the potential size of the problem. In states where a large proportion of the population is more than sixty-five years of age, their lack of prescription drug coverage is likely to be more salient than in states with relatively more youthful populations. Seniors are also active in lobbying for health care benefits for themselves. Thus, we expect the size of the senior population to be positively related to the dependent variables not just through its impact on public opinion but also as an indicator of latent support for interest organizations supporting senior causes. The states' senior populations ranged from 18.1 percent in Florida to 5.6 percent in Alaska in 1999.

The impact of market structure. But SPAPs are not the only way to address high drug prices. HMOs are also designed to hold down the costs of medical care, including limiting the costs of prescription drugs by use of a formulary, market leverage, and in some cases limitations on patients. Thus, their significant presence in a state is expected by some to help drive down drug prices overall. Even if they do not do so, HMOs still constitute a rival approach to controlling high drug costs for their members, which should reduce the pressure on legislators to support SPAPs and render already-established programs less generous (the HMO policy substitution effect).

Conversely, HMOs are also potentially influential—if often latent—interest organizations that tend to support innovative health policies (the

HMO policy facilitation effect), leading to a positive prediction for adoption of SPAPs. For example, Volden (2006) found that innovative elements of the CHIP program diffused across states with similar HMO structures. And Satterthwaite (2002) found that states with a long history of HMOs were more likely to use managed care models in their Medicaid programs. We examine whether the HMO policy substitution or facilitation effect is dominant. We measure HMO presence with the proportion of the population enrolled in HMOs.[14]

VARIABLE SET THREE: STATE RESOURCE CAPACITY

In order to take action on public problems, states must also have the capacity to respond to them. We propose two variables to capture the concept of state wealth, a staple of innovation studies. Researchers routinely find that wealthier states are more likely to innovate, and we expect the same here for a redistributive program. Indeed, Grogan (1993) has argued that with respect to health care *only* relatively wealthy states can innovate. And Satterthwaite (2002) found that wealthy states were more likely to adopt managed care models in their Medicaid programs.

The impact of gross state product. We use two measures of wealth; one is a long-term measure, and the other a short-term measure. The long-term indicator is per capita gross state product (GSP), which measures the overall wealth of the state. The higher the GSP per person, the more likely a state will be to adopt, expand, and make more generous a new program such as a SPAP. This is because, according to innovation theory, wealthy states have slack resources. However, just because states are wealthy it does not mean they automatically choose to tax themselves or to spend general revenues on redistributive policies; politics is also involved.

The impact of a change in state revenues. So we also use a short-term measure, the annual percentage change in total state revenues. This reflects the amount a state actually has chosen to spend and whether the trajectory is going upward or downward. New and more generous SPAPs are more likely to be adopted in states with growing revenue bases; when state revenues decline, fewer new programs will be adopted.

VARIABLE SET FOUR: POLITICAL CONSIDERATIONS

A fourth set of factors addresses the role of politics. At the most global level, drug assistance programs entail a transfer of resources from taxpayers to low-income seniors. It is plausible to expect, then, that states with more liberal citizens and leaders will be more supportive of such policies than states with more conservative citizens and leaders. In general, the Democratic Party is more populated by liberals and the Republican Party by conservatives (Erikson, Wright, and McIver 1993), so party control can be expected to determine which kinds of policies are enacted. And party competition seems to make political parties more attentive to their constituents.

Citizen ideology. A variety of measures of political ideology have been employed in studies of state Medicaid policy; their findings are likely to be applicable to an analysis of SPAPs. Barrilleaux and Miller (1988) measured ideology with ADA scores of state congressional delegations and found support for the ideology hypothesis, as did Grogan (1994) who measured ideology by Elazar's political culture scores. However, Kousser (2002) found that ideology as measured by Erikson, Wright, and McIver (1993) had little influence on the discretionary portion of state Medicaid policy. We believe that the Erikson and colleagues' measure of citizen ideology is the best measure of citizen preferences about the scope of government. Liberal states should more readily adopt, expand, and have more generous pharmacy assistance programs.

Party control. Another in the set of political hypotheses addresses partisan determinants of innovation. We expect states with Democratic governors and legislatures will be more likely to adopt and maintain more generous assistance programs. Kousser's (2002) analysis of the discretionary portion of Medicaid found Democratic control of the legislature to be an important predictor of states' generosity in optional spending. And indeed, Democratic control of the institutions of government is often associated with the adoption of new social spending programs whereas Republican control is not. Thus we expect Democrats to be more supportive of SPAPs than Republicans.

Party control has been measured in a variety of ways over the years: the proportion of Democrats or Republicans in each house, the proportion of Democrats/Republicans in the two chambers combined, the legislative partisan proportions combined with the gubernatorial measure of party control, and so on. We chose to measure Democratic control of the governorship in a streamlined and straightforward way, with a dichotomous variable, coded 1 for Democrats and 0 for Republicans. To reduce problems of collinearity, we use a single measure of Democratic control of the legislature: the average of two dichotomous variables indicating Democratic control of the lower and upper chambers.[15] Again, Democratic control of a legislative chamber is coded 1 and Republican control is coded 0; chambers with split party control are coded as 0.5. Thus, on either the gubernatorial or legislative party control measures we expect a positive coefficient signifying Democrats' control of the institutions of government that adopt, expand, and create more generous SPAPs.

Party competition. The last political variable is interparty competition, a measure used by some but by no means all health policy researchers. But in closely related research on Medicaid, Pracht (2007) found that competition between the two major political parties played a significant role: The closer the competition between the two major parties, the higher the enrollment in Medicaid managed care plans. Similarly, we expect that the more evenly competition is divided between the two political parties, the higher the likelihood of enrolling seniors in newly created SPAPs that will later be revised and made more generous. This is because the more closely partisan the contest, the more parties are likely to make policy appeals to the electorate and to offer new programs aimed at the median voter. We measure interparty competition by using the standard measure—the folded Ranney Index. Given the coding on this index, high values for it indicate relatively high levels of interparty competition, and thus we expect more adoptions, more revisions, and more generosity to be positively correlated with the index.

VARIABLE SET FIVE: PROGRAM HISTORY

The penultimate set of hypotheses is less concerned with innovation per se than with what happens once programs are implemented. That is, the ensuing program history might make program revision more or less likely and might enhance or diminish the generosity of programs. One substantial body of literature suggests that there is typically pressure to expand benefits and coverage when redistributive programs are revised as supporters seek larger coalitions to secure passage (Meier and Copeland 1984). This explanation leads to later adopters of an innovation having more extensive policies than earlier adopters (Boehmke and Witmer 2004; Glick and Hays 1991). And by the same logic, programs that have been revised should be more generous than those that have not. Yet programs that were very generous to begin with must face something of a ceiling effect in terms of further expansion of benefits. There should be less need to expand these programs in the future. And Kim and Jennings (2012) found that later adopters of Medicaid managed care tended to implement less extensive programs than earlier adopters, perhaps due to social learning. We address elements of program history with four variables.

Program age indicator. The first is a dichotomous variable indicating whether a state adopted a prescription drug program before 1990. These early adopters had no need to adopt a new program during the 1990s. Thus, we stipulate their adoption in the models testing hypotheses about the adoption dependent variable while retaining these cases in models of program expansion and generosity.

Age of program in years. Indeed, because these early adopters' programs had been in operation for some time, major program revision on their part during the 1990s might be more likely than for more recent adopters. To test this hypothesis, we include in the model of program expansion a measure of the age of a program in years since initially adopted or 1990 if adopted earlier. If programs do become more expansive over time, the age counter should generate a positive estimate in the generosity model. The organizational theory literature offers competing expectations about how the age of a program should influence its generosity and prospects for revision. In organization ecology research, these are often referred to as the "liability of senescence" and "liability of newness" hypotheses (Hannan and Carroll 1992). If the probability of being revised is a constant, then older programs are more likely to be revised. Moreover, older programs may simply become out-of-date, necessitating revision. However, more than a little tinkering might take place as the bugs are worked out in new programs, which suggests that program revision is more likely early on. Similarly, there are conflicting expectations with regard to program age and generosity. We might plausibly expect that older programs will provide more generous provisions because they will have had time to accumulate benefits designed to expand supporting coalitions. But it is equally plausible that younger programs will be more generous because they start by building on the shoulders of those that have already been established in other states.

Program expansion. Although program expansion is a dependent variable in one model, it is also employed as an independent variable in the generosity model. That is, revision could render drug assistance programs more (or less) generous.

Program generosity. Fourth, to assess whether the initial generosity of a program makes it more (or less) likely that it will be later revised, we include in the expansion model an indicator of the generosity of the initial version of a program.

VARIABLE SET SIX: EXTERNAL INFLUENCES

We now discuss the two external influences we examined—horizontal diffusion, measured by the policies of neighboring states; and the vertical diffusion hypothesis.

The impact of neighbors' programs. The fact that neighboring states have SPAP policies should make such policies more attractive to voters and to policymakers. Various researchers, from Walker (1969) to Canon and Baum (1981) to Berry and Berry (1990), have found regional diffusion effects to be important in explaining the spread of innovations. In the health arena closest to pharmacy assistance, Satterthwaite (2002), Miller (2006), Kim and Jennings (2012), and Grogan (1994) have found that horizontal diffusion operated in the aspects of the Medicaid programs they studied. Thus we expect that public support for prescription assistance will be greater in states neighboring others that have already adopted such programs. We measure neighbors' policy activity by the proportion of neighboring states that have already adopted an SPAP.[16]

The impact of vertical diffusion. Diffusion from the top down is the other external influence we explore. State policymakers do not always turn to their geographic neighbors for information but rather may take their cues from national policy developments. These developments could include discussions and debates in Washington, policy activity in noncontiguous states, and independent media framing efforts that put issues on the policy agenda. We expect that time-pressed officials will find following national developments in the media to be the easiest route, and thus we develop an index of newspaper attention to the issue of pharmacy assistance for seniors. Both Karch (2007) and Lamothe (2005) have found similar indices to be important in explaining policy innovations. Specifically, we performed a Lexis/Nexis search of all newspapers in their database using the keywords "senior citizens" + "prescription drugs." We conducted this search for the extended period from 1975, when the first SPAP law was enacted, to 2001, when our study ends, because there was no reason to restrict this search to just the 1990–2001 period. As shown in figure 3.2, the number of stories on this topic was small until 1998 and 1999, when there were spikes; then the next year, 2000, the number of stories doubled, only to fall back to the recent spike level in the following year. The correlation of this time series tracks quite well the adoption of laws time series shown in figure 3.1. The correlation of the two series, when the variable newspaper stories is lagged as it is in the model, is a robust +.82, suggesting that when we include vertical diffusion in the multivariate model it will have explanatory power.

Testing the Hypotheses

We now turn to testing of the hypotheses, using the variables described above and the 1990–2001 data set for state pharmacy assistance programs.

Figure 3.2 Number of Newspaper Stories on Pharmaceutical Assistance for Seniors, 1975–2001

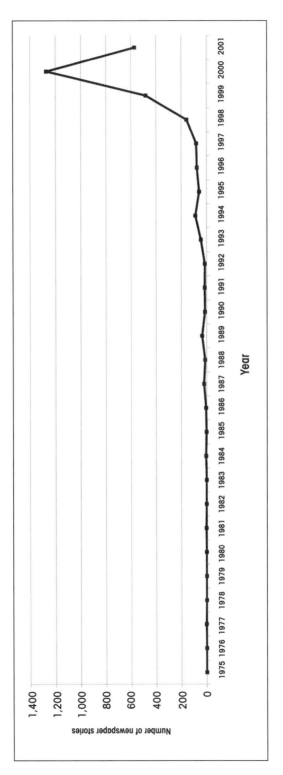

Source: Results of Lexis/Nexis search by the authors.

Estimation

We estimate the models with Heckman probit and Heckman maximum likelihood regression models.[17] Heckman models allow us to test whether there is any selection bias in moving from the sample used to test hypotheses about the adoption of prescription drug programs to the samples used to test models of program revision and generosity. That is, some of the variables that determine whether a state adopts a drug program are plausibly correlated with some of the variables that determine how generous that program is and the likelihood of its being revised. In such cases, the estimates of the generosity and expansion models might be biased and inefficient (Grier, Munger, and Roberts 1994). It must be noted, however, that Heckman models are themselves notoriously fickle. Even modest collinearity problems can make them unstable, even in the face of what seem like minor specification changes. We examined multiple specifications. In doing so, we did not resolve all stability problems. We will see that identically specified selection models of program adoption coupled, respectively, to the program expansion and generosity models and using identically measured variables produced slightly different coefficients. Still, the specifications underlying our results are the most stable of those we examined, in the sense that their estimates are in broad substantive agreement with those generated using several other estimation techniques commonly employed in the innovation literature. Last, all the models employ robust standard errors clustered on states.

Findings

The models are presented in table 3.1. The first pair of models includes a probit selection model examining the determinants of drug program adoption and a probit model assessing the hypotheses on program revision. The second pair of models includes a nearly identical probit selection model of program adoption and its accompanying regression model on the generosity of prescription drug programs.[18] The two selection models generate slightly different estimates.

Let us begin with our key variables of concern, the set of interest organization variables. Looking at the adoption of SPAPs in either Model 1 or Model 2, it is clear that organized interests in the health sector have little to no influence over the adoption of these innovations, with the exception of the percent AARP membership in the state. Evidently, neither the organized proponents nor the opponents registered to lobby have an edge in the struggle over adding SPAPs to state budgets. Neither the total number of health interests nor the percentage of those that were for-profit had an impact on this policy innovation. Only the

Table 3.1 Heckman Estimates of Adoption, Revision, and Generosity of State Pharmaceutical Assistance Programs, Time Series 1990–2001 (n = 600)

	Model 1		Model 2	
	Adoption (Probit)	Expansion (Probit)	Adoption (Probit)	Generosity (OLS)
Interest organization variables				
Estimated no. of health interests	−.003	.003	−.003	−.017***
	(−0.43)	(3.76)	(−0.41)	(−3.66)
Estimated percentage of drug interests	−.001	.105***	.068	−.399
	(−0.00)	(3.87)	(0.35)	(−3.01)
Estimated percentage of advocacy interests	−.376	−.289	−.714	1.24**
	(−0.83)	(−3.31)	(−1.38)	(2.18)
Estimated percentage of health finance interests	−.231	−.165##	−.519	.556
	(−0.61)	(−2.25)	(−1.26)	(1.57)
Percentage of AARP members	.041*	.014**	.064**	−.055
	(1.39)	(2.03)	(1.73)	(−2.68)
Percentage of for-profit interests	.117	−.006	.175	.225
	(2.00)	(−0.34)	(2.80)	(4.44)
Policy diffusion variables				
Lagged no. of newspaper stories	.001***	.0002*	.001***	−.000
	(2.91)	(1.34)	(2.79)	(−1.03)
Lagged percentage of neighbor adoptions	−1.38	.078	−1.68	−1.11
	(−1.74)	(0.35)	(−2.11)	(−1.44)
Program variables				
Pre-1990 adoption	11.51***	–	13.57***	–
	(7.93)		(9.70)	
Program age	–	−.0003***	–	.0002
		(−5.08)		(0.94)
Initial generosity	–	.058**	–	–
		(1.95)		
Program revision	–	-	–	1.41***

Table 3.1 (continued)

Political variables				
Opinion liberalism	4.48**	.418	7.33***	2.77*
	(2.25)	(0.71)	(3.28)	(1.60)
Folded Ranney index	8.09***	−.240	9.58***	0.963
	(2.74)	(−0.53)	(3.03)	(0.49)
Democratic governor	−.653	.143**	−.634	−.399
	(−2.00)	(1.82)	(−2.09)	(−1.49)
Democratic legislature	.268	.149*	.074	−.253
	(0.69)	(1.27)	(0.21)	(−0.65)
Capacity variables				
Per capita GSP	.0002***	−.000	.0002***	.0001*
	(3.53)	(−0.14)	(3.63)	(1.49)
Percentage annual change in state revenue	.168**	−.048	.211***	−.131
	(2.28)	(−1.38)	(2.85)	(−1.18)
Problem environment variables				
Lagged per capita drug costs	−.001	−.001	−.002	.004
	(−0.30)	(−0.53)	(−0.50)	(1.01)
Lagged HMO penetration	−3.55**	−1.46**	−5.41**	2.07
	(−1.66)	(−1.78)	(−2.22)	(0.88)
Lagged percentage of population > 65	.542***	.045**	.706***	−.267
	(3.57)	(1.65)	(3.12)	(−1.32)
Constant	−24.55###	3.26##	−27.68###	−23.26##
	(−2.53)	(1.99)	(−2.71)	(−2.09)
Wald chi-square	847.20		596.18	
Prob > chi-square	0.00		0.00	
Wald test of independent equations	2.92		15.89	
Prob > chi-square	0.09		0.000	

Note: Coefficients are standardized; z statistics in parentheses.

* $p < 0.10$, ** $p < 0.05$, *** $p < 0.01$, one-tailed test with robust standard errors clustered on states.

# $p < 0.10$, ## $p < 0.05$, ### $p < 0.01$, two-tailed test with robust standard errors clustered on states.

Source: Calculated by the authors.

mobilization of senior citizens into AARP chapters and presumably the subsequent lobbying activities of those state chapters made a difference in increasing the number of SPAP adoptions.

The picture changes when we look at the expansion of existing SPAPs in the second column of model 1. There, in addition to AARP membership being a significant variable, the proportion of pharmaceutical interests was positive, and the percentage of health finance interests was negative, using a two-tailed test. Evidently, health plans, health business services, employer health coalitions, and insurance firms do not see the expansion of SPAPs as consistent with their self-interest, as indicated by the negative sign on the coefficient. But pharmacy interests deem an expansion of the number of seniors who can buy drugs to be in their business interest, as suggested by the positive sign on its coefficient. Likewise, AARP's positive and significant coefficient means that greater AARP membership concentration within a state provides some of the lobbying clout needed to expand existing pharmacy programs.

Finally, when we try to explain the programmatic generosity of SPAPs, the number of health interests is a negative predictor, such that we might think policy gridlock was being produced on the mere consideration of making these programs more generous. The proportion of advocacy interests among groups registered to lobby had a positive and significant impact on the generosity of SPAPs. The key variable among supportive organized interests is the proportion of health advocacy interests, in contrast to the key variable among opponents, which is the number of health interests stalemating the enhancement of program generosity. This was the only dimension of pharmacy assistance on which AARP membership did not make a difference. Concentration of AARP membership did not lead to more lobbying by their organization in support of enhanced generosity for existing programs. It seems, then, that organized interests have little impact on program adoption but have a great deal more to say about program revision and generosity.

What about political variables? Political ideology—as measured by the Wright, Erickson, and McIver (1993) scale—is positively and significantly related to the adoption of SPAPs in both model 1 and model 2 of table 3.1. What citizens think about the scope of government evidently matters to policymakers as they debate establishing this new role for government. The more a state's citizens believe in a broader scope for government and adopt a liberal position, the more likely it is that state pharmacy assistance programs will be enacted in response to those public preferences.

In terms of party control of the institutions of government, having a Democratic governor or legislature is not helpful in adopting these programs, contrary to our predictions. The gubernatorial variable even carries a negative sign. However, the variable of interparty competition is consistently and positively predictive of the adoption of these laws. Where there are close races between the two political parties, the more likely it is that SPAPs will be adopted. This is what happened at the federal level: After the 2000 election both political parties were competing to deliver better drug coverage to seniors on Medicare. In sum, the likelihood of SPAP adoption is enhanced by citizen ideology being in the liberal direction and by relatively even competition between the two parties.

Looking at program expansion, the picture changes so that both the Democratic governor and legislature are keys to expanding pharmacy assistance programs. Both institutions of governments carry positive and significant coefficients, meaning that when Democrats control the institutions of policymaking, they are able to use them to expand the benefits and coverage of redistributive programs consonant with their base constituency. Moving onto explaining generosity, the only political variable that is of any significance is public opinion liberalism, which is modestly significant and positive. Where states score high in citizen liberalism, state policymakers are more likely to enact their preferences for designing redistributive programs to cover the most people. Otherwise, politics does not have much to do with making SPAPs more (or less) generous after they are initiated.

Next we come to the capacity variables, where we expected that financial resources are necessary for new programs of any kind to be adopted. And indeed, the adoption of SPAPs is positively and significantly related to per capita GSP and to change in state revenue. Where states are relatively well off, leaders are more likely to enact legislation to spend money on new programs; similarly, where the annual budget trend is in the positive direction, state policymakers are more liable to adopt programs that commit financial resources as SPAPs do. Measures of state wealth did not have any discernible impact on program revisions. The models suggest that states expand their SPAPs without regard to their level of wealth. And only per capita GSP had a modest, positive impact on programmatic generosity; the short-term measure of state wealth—annual changes in state revenue—was unrelated to program generosity. Clearly, wealth matters more in getting the SPAP initiated than in the later phases of the program.

Now we examine the variables that measure need for the pharmacy assistance program and other aspects of the problem environment. The increasing cost of drugs does not seem to be a program driver; it in fact registered a negative coefficient, though not a significant one, opposite from our prediction for adoptions. What did make a difference was the size of the senior population: The higher the percentage of the population over the age of sixty-five years, the more likely it was that a SPAP was adopted. This coefficient was strongly positive. The effect of HMO penetration was significant, though not quite as strong, and in the negative direction, meaning that more SPAPs were adopted in states with few HMO members. This finding is consistent with a substitution effect for HMOs. It implies that HMOs represent an alternative or substitute approach to addressing issues of high drug costs for their members that should, in turn, reduce the public pressure on legislators to enact SPAPs.

Turning to the program expansion phase, HMO penetration continues to have a substitution effect, as suggested by its negative and significant coefficient. The more concentrated the presence of HMOs in a state, the less likely it is that states will expand their existing programs. The relative size of the senior population demonstrates a significant positive coefficient, so that states with more seniors also do more revising of their programs. With respect to program generosity, none of the need variables governs programmatic generosity. However, two of the three need variables are a pretty potent explanation for initial policy adoption in pharmacy assistance.

Our next set of variables includes the program variables that are unique to this model. They are introduced because we had to truncate the sample and omit some years of adoption. The first variable is pre-1990 adoption, which reflects only our stipulation that these states adopted programs before our sample period. But for program age in years, we learn that leader states are less likely to expand these older programs as compared with new programs, which are more likely to be revised; this coefficient is negative and highly significant. Such a pattern suggests that the "liability of newness" is operating here. Probably the bugs are being worked out in these new programs, indicating a necessity for tinkering, leading to program revision to solve the problems. Also, a program's initial level of generosity is positively and significantly related to expansion, meaning that the programs that are more generous to begin with are the ones more likely to be expanded. Perhaps they are found in states with relatively greater commitments to their seniors. And looking at the generosity model, the only relationship here is with program revision: The coefficient is highly significant and positive, indicating that when programs are revised, they become more generous programmatically. This result reinforces our view that most of the program revisions were in effect program expansions providing more generous benefits to recipients.

Finally, we look at the set of policy diffusion variables that may have an impact on the adoption, expansion, and generosity of SPAPs. First, we examine horizontal diffusion where policy activity by one's neighbors may make adoption more likely. That did not happen here; in fact, the coefficient has a negative sign, though insignificant, across three measures of SPAP policy. Thus, interstate diffusion is not an explanation. Second, we examine the number of newspaper stories on seniors and drug costs as a proxy for national developments that might be affecting states. These lagged coefficients are strong and positive for the adoption of SPAPs and modestly significant and positive for their further expansion, but not related to their generosity. The strong positive coefficients indicate that state policymakers may be taking cues from national discussion of and activity on pharmacy assistance policies and programs.

Summarizing Findings about the Three Models

To summarize our findings about each of the models, the politics of adoption of pharmacy assistance programs is in general not the politics of organized interests. This is certainly not what we expected to find after watching prescription drugs being added to the Medicare program in Congress over its several cycles, where it was indeed the politics of special interests. At the state level, established health interests made little impact one way or the other. The only organized interest of moderate significance was the large membership-based AARP organization, which boosted the chances that states would enact SPAPs. Nor was the politics of SPAP adoption influenced by governmental institutions such as the state legislature or the governor, neither of which made a statistically discernible difference. Rather, opinion liberalism and close interparty competition were the two mechanisms translating citizen support for adoption of pharmacy assistance programs; both had sizable positive coefficients as predicted.

Wealth, both in the long term and in the short term, mattered. Wealthier states and states where the revenues were trending upward were more likely to adopt SPAPs, again as predicted. We were surprised that the rise in drug costs did not matter as part of the proximate problem environment, but as predicted the proportionate size of the senior population did matter for adoption. Also HMO penetration had a substitution effect, meaning that managed care might have operated as an alternative way to manage pharmacy costs. Finally, national diffusion in the form of newspapers' attention to the issue increased adoption, as predicted, but state-to-state diffusion had no effect.

Next we summarize the findings for the model of program revision. Here organized interests had more impact: AARP still had its positive impact, but the percentage of drug interests was also positive and highly significant. Evidently once SPAPs get going, pharmaceutical manufacturers like the programs and want to expand them to enroll more people. However, the percentage of health finance interests, which we indicated could go either way on expansion, evidently is swayed too much by arguments about the costs of the SPAPs and who will pay for them. Its coefficient is negatively signed and significant in a two-tailed test. Democratic control of the institutions of state government now becomes critical for program expansion; both the governor and legislature had positive and significant coefficients. Oddly state capacity did not seem to matter. Perhaps the state's policymakers had figured out that the initial program was affordable and that tinkering with it would not break the bank. Revising the programs did seem to grow out of one kind of need—the size of the senior population was positively and significantly related to program revision, though drug costs were not a factor. Lagged HMO penetration had a negative and significant coefficient at the .05 level for program revision, again suggesting the substitution effect. Horizontal diffusion did not play a role in program revision, though national diffusion played a positive and significant role. Unique program variables indicated that newer programs were much more likely to be revised, and initially more generous programs were more likely to be revised. Overall, program revision and expansion was more the province of organized interests than was adoption of the same programs. Supportive interests ally with Democrats controlling the institutions of government to enact the revisions, and they are sensitive to the needs of constituents such as seniors.

Finally, we can summarize the results for the generosity model, recalling that we are talking about programmatic elements of generosity, not financial benefits. The politics of organized interests plays out in two ways in generosity. First, the greater the number of health interests in a state, the lower the generosity of the program. This coefficient is negative and highly significant. Second, the higher the percentage of advocacy interests, the more likely that states will have generous programs. None of the other interest-based measures are significant. Politics does not matter much. The only political variable that is significant is public opinion liberalism, and that is modestly so ($p < .10$) in the positive direction. In terms of state capacity, only per capita GSP matters. Its coefficient is positive, as predicted, but significant only at the $p < .10$ level. None of the three problem environment or need variables is important to the explanation for generosity. Neither is policy diffusion of either kind. Finally, looking at the unique program variables, only program revision is significant and highly so in the positive direction, meaning that the more programs are revised, the more generous they become. Overall, the generosity of SPAPs is not as well explained by our model as were their adoption and revision.

Among the different sets of variables, however, organized interests make the greatest contribution to the explanation, with two highly significant coefficients.

Conclusion

Several conclusions seem justified about the politics of state pharmacy assistance programs. First, our results suggest that the balance of democratic and interest organization influences on public policy varies markedly across the program adoption, expansion, and generosity stages. Program adoption seems to be the venue in which the democratic influences of close interparty competition and liberal public preferences hold the most sway, though these preferences seem not to have been expressed through election of Democratic governors and legislatures. States with greater capacity and more need as measured by more seniors were more likely to adopt prescription drug policies. Organized interests certainly play a key role in the democratic process via articulating need, capacity, and preferences. But in sharp contrast to the canonical story of the Medicare Modernization Act being a giant pork barrel for health industry interests, we found little evidence that the density of health interests and both their diversity and that of the overall interest system had any additional independent impact on the likelihood of a state adopting a prescription drug program. The only interest group that seems to have made a difference is AARP, which was working to improve the lives of low-income seniors.

Rather, organized interests seem more at home when revising public policies, probably a lower-salience activity. Indeed, the pattern of results across the adoption, revision, and generosity models suggests that the politics of revision is often about fine-tuning public policies so as to better satisfy the needs of special interests, usually in the context of expanding a program. Program expansion occurred in states with a high proportion of drug interests, presumably because they desired more customers who could afford to purchase their products. Also, such states were characterized by having proportionately more AARP members and fewer health finance interests. Generosity of programs was advanced by having fewer health interests lobbying overall and by having relatively more advocacy interests.

However, "democratic" electoral and public preference constraints are also at play in the process of pharmacy program revision and generosity. Putting Democrats in control of the governorship and the state legislature increases the likelihood of revising the original law. Having more seniors over the age of sixty-five years also increases the probability that a state will expand their original programs. Program generosity was enhanced by liberal public preferences and state wealth, as measured by per capita GSP.

Perhaps least controversially, program history and context matter. The newness of a state's prescription drug program and its initial generosity influence its rate of expansion, while whether it has been revised improves its generosity. Although we had competing expectations about the role of HMOs in holding down drug costs, our results suggest that managed care organizations are best viewed as an element of context. HMOs constitute an independent means of addressing drug costs. When HMO penetration is extensive, states seem less inclined to support prescription drug policies; witness California, as perhaps the most surprising state without a prescription assistance program.[19] But one element of context that does not seem to matter, or at least not so in the manner commonly expected in the literature on policy diffusion, concerns neighbors' adoption of similar programs. The proportion of neighboring states with drug assistance programs was not significantly related to program adoption, generosity, or program expansion. But diffusion from a different source was certainly operating in the adoption of this innovation, and that was diffusion from national media sources. Evidently, the peak year of adoption, 2001, can be traced in part to the print media's focus on coverage of the drug cost issue in 2000, especially during the presidential election campaign, when candidates Bush and Gore offered competing versions of how to help seniors with their drug costs. In 2001 alone, six states adopted new SPAPs, and seven expanded existing programs.

Of particular importance, our results do not indicate that organized interests always win or that democratic influences are unimportant in revising and expanding prescription drug programs. When need is high, as measured by the relative size of the senior population, and when programs are younger and initially more generous, expansion is likely to happen. And it is more likely to happen when the Democrats control both institutions of state government. Moreover, the politics of organized interests is not always a game of good guys versus bad guys, *with the bad guys always winning*. As Smith (2000) noted, the "bad" guys are especially vulnerable when they are united against strong public preferences. Faced with choosing between the preferences of their constituents and those of organized interests, politicians have very strong incentives to support their constituents. Instead, organized interests are far more effective when pursuing narrow policies falling below the radar of public opinion and without opposition from other organized interests. Prescription drug policy seems to fit Smith's third and intermediate category of interest conflict, in which two or more interest sectors are pitted against each other. In our case, the proportion of organizations representing drug interests is positively related to revision as is the AARP membership base, while higher relative representation by health finance interests seems to reduce the chances that the initial form of a state's drug policy will be altered. Which side wins depends, of course, on the specific configuration of a state's interest system. Also the outcome is influenced by the market structure in the state, with extensive HMO penetration reducing program expansion.

Finally, the generosity of prescription drug programs is determined by the frequency and direction of program revisions. It is not surprising, then, that our results indicate that generosity is influenced both by the democratic forces of capacity and public preferences and by competition among organized interests with a stake in public policy. This summary finding is, of course, quite consistent with neopluralist assessments of the balance of democratic and nondemocratic forces in American politics (McFarland 2004; Lowery and Gray 2004b). It is far less consistent, however, with the consensus interpretation of the politics of health care springing from President Bush's addition of a pharmacy benefit to Medicare and his further efforts to "modernize" it. That episode in American history was summed up as the purchase of a benefit at the expense of a wide array of pork barrel benefits for providers, insurance companies, and pharmaceutical manufacturers (Heaney 2006, 929). If the states' experiences with prescription drug programs tell us anything, it is that the politics of state health care is far more complex, far more interesting, and potentially far more optimistic than the national story.

At this point in our story the future of state pharmacy assistance programs depends upon how they function in concert with the national Medicare program as the ACA begins to fill in the doughnut hole in Part D. How will federal officials work with state officials to ensure that low-income seniors enroll in Medicare Part D and take advantage of the states' wraparound programs that help bridge the drug coverage gap? The evidence of federal officials learning from the states when contemplating the MMA was nonexistent, according to Weissert and Scheller (2008): Few state representatives testified before Congress at the time. Those who did testify urged that Congress recognize the valuable lessons learned by the states in making coverage decisions, negotiating rates (which Congress expressly forbids Medicare to do), and contracting with pharmacy benefits managers. Congress and the Bush administration passed up this chance to learn from the states in 2003; now we will see if the Obama administration views the states as allies and seeks to build upon their record in the administration of pharmacy assistance.

Notes

1. Hall and Van Houweling (2006) state that the private-sector health industry spent $100 million in 2003, but that the next year they spent even more.

2. At the time to get prescription drug coverage seniors paid $35 per month, after meeting a $250 deductible; then Medicare paid 75 percent of their drug costs up to $2,250 per year. Then the government paid nothing until the senior has paid $3,600 out of pocket; at that point 95 percent of drug costs were covered by the government. Low-income seniors get additional financial help from the government. For details on the effects of the "doughnut hole," see Rosenthal (2004).

3. High-income seniors (those with incomes above $100,000) pay extra for premiums for Part B of Medicare.

4. Only thirty-one of the thirty-four states had enacted the pharmacy benefit by 2001 and are thus in our data set, which covers the study period 1990–2001.

5. Additional states have programs that only provide discounts to eligible citizens.

6. Full information on the structure of state interest populations—as measured by lobby registration data—is available for only a limited number of years: 1980, 1990, 1997, 1998, and 1999. There are considerable difficulties in relying on these data much past 2001 given that we would be extrapolating well beyond our data on interest organizations. Even more problematic is the period from 1980 to 1990, when state interest systems doubled in size. In the states for which we have complete data, this pattern of growth included population booms and busts (Brasher, Lowery, and Gray 1999). Thus, we have only the endpoints and beginning points of a period of very dynamic growth. We think that it is inappropriate to make overly generous assumptions about annual values of lobby registrations for this very dynamic period of growth. Although lobby registrations still grew across the states in the 1990s, the available evidence (Brasher, Lowery, and Gray 1990; Wolak, Lowery, and Gray 2001) indicates that growth during the 1990s was more incremental in character.

7. We tried to examine the earlier period, using data from 1980 onward and a less valid measure of the number of organized interests in 1980 than we employ here. Using this less valid measure over the longer time period from 1980 to 2001 and over the truncated period from 1990 to 2001 examined here generated very similar results. Thus, we do not think that the shortened period per se influences our findings. Problems with the validity of the interest group measures for the earlier period suggest that these models may well not be telling us the full story of their role in policy adoptions. And there are other good reasons to suspect that the specification employed here is less appropriate for the earlier period and for the most recent period from 2001 onward. In both the more routine politics of health care in the 1980s and the stringent fiscal conditions following 2001, budgetary issues are plausibly more important in determining state policy adoptions

than they were during the 1990s. And since 2003 the mandates of Medicare Part D have affected the states, especially the requirement that states fund most of the pharmacy expenses of the so-called dual eligibles, those eligible for both Medicaid and Medicare. A fuller specification encompassing the full period should, therefore, address a different set of determinants associated with the fiscal conditions of the states. However, these can essentially be treated as temporal constants for the period examined here, except insofar as we control for differences in the wealth of the states. During the 1990s there was far more variation in wealth across the states than across time within states, although our wealth measure (per capita gross state product) controls for both.

8. Although a number of states made additional revisions in their programs after 2001, before then, only one state had adopted a second significant revision of its prescription drug policy—Vermont in 2000. With only a 2000 and a 2001 observation on but one state, we focus only on the first major revision of drug policies.

9. The procedures used to code the state lobby registration data have been described more fully elsewhere (Gray and Lowery 2001). Briefly, however, lobby registration lists were gathered by mail or Web page from state agencies responsible for their maintenance. After purging the lists of state agencies in states requiring their registration, organizations registered to lobby—rather than individual lobbyists—were coded by interest content (twenty-six guilds of substantive interests) using directories of organizations and associations and the Web pages of individual organizations. The senior author then examined the coding assignments with discrepancies resolved via discussion between the two people. There was little difficulty in assigning most substantive codes. For example, only 1.58 percent of the 35,771 organizational lobby registrations in 1997 could not be coded by type or substantive interest. Fortunately, previous work indicates that the stringency of state lobbying registration requirements has little impact on the density (Lowery and Gray 1994, 1997) and diversity (Gray and Lowery 1998b) of state interest communities.

10. Only thirty-one organizations in the 1999 health population could not be so coded. The largest health subguilds, constituting half of all health registrations, were seven categories providing direct patient care.

11. The 1999 and 2000 data on AARP membership were not available and were interpolated from each state with data from 1998 and 2001. This should not constitute a serious problem given that the far larger source of variation in this measure is across states rather than across time. We also examined the interaction of the size of the senior population, which we include as a need variable, and the AARP proportion included in the model as an organized interest variable. Surprisingly, the two variables were negatively, if weakly, correlated ($r = 0.198$). Thus, they are indeed measuring different things. But when both were included in the models with their interaction, few of the coefficients were significant, likely due to high collinearity. Thus, we present the results separately for the two variables.

12. This low percentage was in part likely a function of California having the highest proportion of residents in HMOs and a large enough population to exert market leverage.

13. The simple correlation of the 1990 and 1998 cross-sectional drug cost measures is 0.796.

14. Data on HMO penetration was not available for 1992. Therefore, this value is interpolated.

15. Although there is neither a house nor house elections in Nebraska, nor partisanship, the unicameral state is retained in the sample. Nebraska's legislative election dummy reflects only the Senate. The partisan value of Nebraska's legislature is set at 0.5, as are all chambers with split party control.

16. Neighboring states are defined by Berry and Berry (1990, 412).

17. Given their growing prevalence since Berry and Berry (1990), we first examined an event history model. Unfortunately, the data requirements of these models are substantial, whereas our individual time series are only eleven years in length. Moreover, it is not clear that program adoption is an "event" as it is usually conceptualized in event history models. The generosity variable is measured at the interval level. And even the adoption variable is something less than temporally discrete. As we have noted, four states suspended their prescription drug programs in recent years, albeit outside our truncated sample of time. And speaking of truncation, our time series are both left and right censured. Though none of these problems individually precludes the use of event history analysis, they certainly make it very difficult to generate any discernible estimates when taken together. One alternative is treating the data as a simple pooled cross-section time-series design and employing a least-squares dummy variable (LSDV) approach to control for pooling-induced heteroscedasticity. Unfortunately, the LSDV would preclude analyzing the variables that are temporal constants, including the density and diversity of for-profit interest organizations. We also examined tobit estimation to address the censuring issue. Unfortunately, neither tobit nor a simple pooled regression using either LSDV or generalized least squares can address the selection bias that might arise from censuring. I.e., we have seen that some of the variables that determine whether a state adopts a drug program are plausibly correlated with some of the variables that determine how generous that program is and the likelihood of its being revised (Grier, Munger, and Roberts 1994). In such cases, the estimates of the generosity and expansion models might be biased and inefficient.

18. Both models include Wald tests of independent equations reported at the bottom of the table. These do not indicate the presence of a severe selection bias, although the second pair of models produced a chi-square value that carries us closer to the borderline of rejecting the null hypothesis of independence.

19. California has only a pharmacy assistance program for genetically handicapped persons.

CHAPTER 4

The Politics of Managing Managed Care

The rise and fall of managed care is one of the most significant stories associated with the politics of health care during the last fifty years. Managed care began from local efforts associated with rural cooperatives in the 1920s and expanded during World War II through the efforts of the industrialist Henry Kaiser. By the late 1960s it had become the preferred option of consumer advocates because of its emphasis on preventive care. At roughly the same time managed care became the preference of business because it controlled health care costs as compared with the existing fee-for-service system. This happy confluence of interests led to a rapid expansion of managed care so that by the end of the twentieth century most Americans with private health insurance received their health care through managed care organizations. But the 1990s were not a happy decade for the managed care industry. Rather than a fortuitous marriage of interests, the strong incentives for health maintenance organizations (HMOs) to control costs came to be perceived by consumers as adverse to their interests in quality of care and in choice of providers. The political response to this changed environment was not long in coming. Beginning in the mid-1990s the states—and the federal government, too—considered a variety of proposals to constrain what were viewed as out-of-control HMOs. The states were successful in imposing a wide variety of regulations on the operation of managed care organizations, including establishing new rights for consumers and enforcing new limits on providers. To proponents, these were necessary correctives in a system that seemed to emphasize controlling costs more than quality of care. To critics, these new regulations seemed to strike at the cost-saving rationale for managed care.

We are, however, less interested in sorting through these conflicting interpretations than in the states' rapid political responses to public perceptions of serious problems with managed care than whether the promise was actually realized. In an era when public policy on health care (and many other issues) was usually described as gridlocked or stalemated at the federal level as a result of intense pressure from organized interests (West, Heith, and Goodwin 1996; Weissert and Weissert 1996; West and Loomis 1999; Jamieson 1994;

Johnson and Broder 1996; Quadagno 2005), many states acted with considerable dispatch in addressing public concerns about HMOs, though some did not. We take advantage of this interstate variation to understand why some governments are able to handle what seem to be intractable policy problems, intractable in a political sense. We are especially interested in the role of organized interests in explaining why some states were very aggressive in regulating HMOs but others were not. From the history of HMOs, the innovation literature, the backlash against managed care, and state responses to that backlash we first extract a number of hypotheses about state regulatory activity in this area. These hypotheses are then tested with data we collected on states' regulatory adoptions during the late 1990s and the early years of the present century. Last, we discuss the findings with special attention to the role of politics in health care. In an ironic turnaround for the much-maligned HMOs, nonprofit health cooperatives were touted during the health reform debates of 2009 as an alternative to a new public option, one that would put consumers in charge of governance and save costs (Sack 2009a). No one seemed to notice that such health cooperatives were the genesis of the beleaguered HMOs, so recently the target of state regulations.

Managed Care Regulation in the States

Before analyzing the states' attempts to regulate managed care, it is useful to have a historical overview of managed care and then to examine the backlash against it that stoked the fires for regulation.

A Short History of Managed Care

Prepaid health insurance originated in the cooperative movement of the 1920s that flourished in America's rural areas. It grew in the postwar period with union support and the leadership in California of Henry Kaiser, who had set up a health plan for his workers during World War II. The first cooperative health plan—a community hospital—was established by the Lebanese physician Dr. Michael Shadid in Elk City, Oklahoma, in 1929. Group health plans that appeared in Washington (1930s), Seattle and New York City (1940s), and Saint Paul (1950s) survived into the next century. Cooperative medicine had to overcome many hurdles, but foremost among them was the opposition of local physicians. In Dr. Shadid's case the county medical society to which he had belonged for twenty years suddenly disbanded and reconstituted itself without him as a member, depriving him of malpractice insurance and making it extremely difficult for him to get patients to come to his hospital

(Group Health 1991, 9). In Washington, the Group Health Association was formed in 1937 as a nonprofit cooperative by employees of a federal agency. The American Medical Association (AMA) prevented referrals to doctors in the fledgling coop and denied them hospital admitting privileges; for such behaviors the AMA was convicted of violating the antitrust act (Starr 1982, 305). Today the Group Health Association in Washington has slightly more than 100,000 members. The antagonism of autonomous physicians to prepaid group practice and consumer governance was to be one of the defining features of the politics of managed care.

In Minnesota the concept of cooperatives was well established as a way of doing business in rural areas. Farmers organized cooperatives to market grain, livestock, milk, eggs, and so on and supplied electricity and telephone service through cooperatives. Yet, even here the idea of health cooperatives was greeted with cries of "socialism" and "communism." Moreover, the organizers faced a barrier that seemed insurmountable: the opinions of three Minnesota attorneys general who stated that the prepaid health cooperatives constituted the corporate practice of medicine, illegal under Minnesota law. So the health reformers began instead by opening the Group Health Mutual insurance company in 1938 to sell hospital insurance (Group Health 1991, 10). As the hospital insurance plan struggled along, the organizers, many of whom were Finns and Swedes from the Iron Range of Minnesota, tried to get a new law passed to make prepaid group medical practices legal, but they had no success. Finally, in 1955 fellow Iron Ranger Miles Lord, later to be a famous federal judge, became attorney general. He ruled that a nonprofit health cooperative would not be considered a corporate practice of medicine. Soon thereafter Group Health Plan was born in Saint Paul; it faced all the challenges of similar plans around the country, such as gaining acceptance by the local medical society but physicians and professors from the University of Minnesota helped to smooth the way with the local medical society. Eventually the plan grew into the 1.2-million-member nonprofit HMO Health Partners, cited in news reports in August 2009 (*NBC Nightly News* 2009) as an example of the health cooperatives that could be established as an alternative to the public option being debated in Congress.

After World War II ended, several other important prepaid group practices sprang up that have also lasted into this century. One is Group Health Cooperative of Puget Sound, which had to face concerted opposition from the local medical community but has grown into a large and successful cooperative, also often singled out in news stories in the summer of 2009 as a model for what health care cooperatives could look like. Also on the West coast, Kaiser decided to bring comprehensive health services to his workers in shipyards and steel mills. In 1942 he set up two Permanente Foundations to run the medical programs, one in the Portland area and the other in Oakland. Because of wartime conditions and because he was providing for his workers, his plans encountered little opposition (Starr 1982, 322). However, when the war ended his workforce shrank and the health plans' enrollment slipped dramatically, so Kaiser decided to open them to the general public. Within ten years his health plan network was expanding, despite having to overcome resistance from the medical community; today Kaiser Permanente is held up as a model of a large HMO that is highly successful. Similarly, the Kaiser network was prominently featured in news stories in August 2009 on health cooperatives that could be emulated in the future. And finally, in New York City the Health Insurance Plan (HIP) had powerful support few other health cooperatives had—the backing of Mayor Fiorello La Guardia. Nonetheless, it took the organizers four years to get the plan up and finally running in 1947 (Starr 1982, 322). Today it remains the largest HMO in New York City and serves patients in three states.

Despite these early struggles, group health plans attracted members and doctors. As long as both patients and providers voluntarily chose their plans, embraced the same philosophy, and could exit the plans, the group practice model worked fairly well. By the early 1970s prepaid group medical cooperatives were still viewed as somewhat subversive, and they tended to attract more liberal to radical doctors and patients. But President Richard Nixon seized upon prepaid group practice as a way to control health care costs and head off the initiation of national health insurance. He welcomed for-profit companies as health plan sponsors and adopted the new term "health maintenance organization" or HMO.[1] There were only thirty such HMOs in operation in the entire country in 1971 (Starr 1982, 396). In response, Congress passed the Health Maintenance Organization Act of 1973, which required employers of more than twenty-five employees to offer at least one HMO option, if there was one in the area, and provided subsidies to such plans. This act marked a critical juncture in the history of prepaid group medicine and spurred the growth of HMOs nationwide. What had been a radical cooperative medical venture for workers, denounced as socialism by its critics, was now a Republican corporate effort to cut costs for employers and install efficiencies in medical practice—a dramatic shift in philosophy. What did not change was the stance of providers. The AMA still voiced opposition, though it was somewhat muted because, after all, these were now Republican HMOs.

By 1982 HMOs had changed the delivery of health care sufficiently for Starr (1982, 429) to declare that corporatization had finally come to medicine, bringing with it a profound loss of physician autonomy. Enrollment increased during the 1980s as the federal government moved Medicare, and especially Medicaid, patients into HMOs. Large businesses made the same choice for their employees. HMOs vertically integrated with hospitals to form new service delivery models, including physician networks working as "preferred provider plans" growing alongside staff-model HMOs. Together termed "managed care," such organizations appeared to achieve significant cost savings over traditional indemnity plans, making them popular with both private and public payers. The proportion of Americans with employer-sponsored coverage in managed care went from 5 percent in 1984 to 85 percent in 1998 (Titlow and Emanuel 1999, 944). Medicaid enrollment in managed care passed the 50 percent mark in 1998 (Oliver 2004, 712). Managed care and the virtues of managed competition became the reigning paradigm in health policy sometime in the early 1990s (Oliver 2004). In 1992 the AMA sent its executive vice president to a conference of the Group Health Association of America to voice the AMA's support for HMOs (Stych 1992). This public recognition was proof that the balance of political power between managed care and fee-for-service physicians had shifted toward managed care.

Backlash against Managed Care

The seed for backlash against managed care came when both patients and doctors were forced into managed care plans against their will. Between 1994 and 1996 private employers shifted from typically offering their workers a choice among health plans to about half offering only a single plan, usually one that emphasized managed care. Often that option was the lowest bid from a for-profit managed care firm—and that option might change every year or two, disrupting the patient–doctor relationship. To stay in business, independent physicians and clinics had to contract with managed care companies. By the early 2000s 88 percent of physicians had contracts with managed care companies; these doctors received, on average, 41 percent of their income from managed care (Casalino 2004, 874). Employers placed millions of unwilling patients into managed care companies not of their own choice, where they were treated by doctors often equally unwilling to be contractually related to the company. Physicians lost professional autonomy—and often income as well—compared with the past; patients in turn were suspicious of decisions made by a cost-conscious insurer, especially one with a for-profit motive. Without the exit option, vocal opposition to managed care began to build.

The backlash against managed care began shortly after the failure of President Clinton's Health Care Security Act in 1994. Clinton's bill had intended to introduce managed competition into the health care marketplace, which would in turn give consumers choices among managed care plans. Deprived of this form of private regulation, consumers and providers turned to the government for relief from managed care bureaucrats. Fifty patient protection measures were introduced in Congress in 1997 and 1998; in early 1999 more than ten comprehensive patient reform bills were introduced (Brown 2001). Though a patient protection bill eventually passed both houses of Congress, it languished and died in conference committee in June 2001. This legislative activity seems to have been motivated by legislators' attentiveness to their constituents and the polls. Managed care emerged as a problem in national polls after 1994, when employee choices among plans vanished. According to Jacobs and Shapiro (1999, 1023), between 1994 and 1998, Americans changed their minds about HMOs, leading 70 percent or more to support consumer protections.

Federal legislators actually were a bit late in responding to this change in public opinion. State policymakers began to turn their attention to "managing" managed care as early as 1994 and 1995, well ahead of the federal government. In the first half of 1996, more than 400 bills to regulate managed care were introduced in state legislatures (Miller 1997, 1102). The first wave of laws was primarily the outcome of physician lobbying. In 1994 any-willing-provider laws were adopted for the first time by seven states. Three states enacted the first bans on "gag" rules the next year. Although the latter is not as significant given that physician behavior can be monitored in ways other than contractual, any-willing-provider laws strike at the heart of managed care and its ability to manage costs and deliver consistent care.

Consumer protection laws followed slightly later, beginning in 1996 and 1997.[2] In 1996 Florida enacted a law setting up the office of ombudsman to assist consumers in filing complaints against managed care companies. In 1997 the state of Texas passed the first liability law, which gave patients the right to sue health plans for malpractice damages. That same year seven states enacted the first laws requiring that patient appeals be reviewed by an independent external reviewer. The possibility that medical decisions will be reviewed and overturned by an outside reviewer—or even worse, from the perspective of HMOs, by a court capable of assessing monetary damages—either shapes up health plan bureaucrats or leads to the practice of defensive and more expensive medicine, depending on one's point of view.

The Texas liability law was eventually overturned by the US Supreme Court in 2004 (*Aetna Health Inc. v Davila*, No. 02-1845). In the *Aetna* case, the Supreme Court clearly ruled in favor of the Employee Retirement Income Security Act (ERISA) preemption, which keeps the regulation of fringe benefits at the federal level. The presence of ERISA complicates enforcement of state health and insurance regulations and has led some critics to charge that state laws are "toothless" (Stone 1999). The US Congress passed ERISA in 1974 to protect workers, specifically their pension plans and other fringe benefits, and to offer employers regulatory consistency across state lines. The states can regulate health insurers who sell individual policies and those who cover state and local governmental employees; they share regulatory authority with the federal government over insurers who operate in the fully insured market (mostly selling to small businesses) (Bovbjerg 2003, 375). Large employers quickly figured out that they could self-insure and come under ERISA, thus escaping state regulation.

Generally speaking, however, the states have keenly protected their regulatory turf. This is especially true in regard to potentially broader federal patient protection proposals that were on political agendas during the latter half of the 1990s and the early 2000s. When the passage of such bills by Congress seemed likely in the spring of 2001, officials of the National Conference of State Legislatures (NCSL) testified that though they welcomed a federal floor of protection, they strongly opposed preemption of state insurance laws and any efforts to expand the ERISA preemption. They especially did not want to have to water down current state regulations in order to meet lower federal standards (Monson 2001).

Even the ERISA preemption, however, may not be as big a roadblock to consumer protection as originally thought. Indeed, in two other cases, the US Supreme Court has overturned the application of the ERISA preemption, leaving states with regulatory leeway. In 2002, in *Rush Prudential HMO v. Moran* (536 US at 383), the Court said that states can require independent external review of coverage denials, even for patients in self-insured plans.[3] The next year, the Court upheld the any-willing-provider law in the case of *Kentucky Association of Health Plans v. Miller* (123 S. Ct. 1471, 1478). Justice Antonin Scalia's majority opinion seemed to signal an all-clear for state regulation of plans, according to Bloche and Studdert (2004).[4] Indeed, managed care organizations seem to have accommodated themselves to state regulation to a considerable degree. Bloche and Studdert (2004, 36), for example, argue that since the late 1990s managed care organizations and their investors have dealt with potential legal conflicts and consumer backlash as a conventional type of business risk. Accordingly, state laws and court cases may have more of an impact through their effects on market actors' perceptions and expectations, rather than through their actual proscriptions. Moreover, HMOs have their own bureaucratic and administrative routines. Once they establish an ombudsman office, an internal appeals process, place report cards on the Internet, and so on, they often extend them across the organization. It would be far too confusing to have report cards posted for members with one kind of insurance coverage and not allow members covered by different insurance plans to read the report cards. For these types of consumer services, HMOs might well prefer to avoid organizational nightmares and the resultant bad publicity arising from an overly legalistic extension of protections to selected classes of patients and not to others.

Given these supportive court cases and the power of bureaucratic routines, we believe that state protection laws are far from "toothless." Indeed, they and the broader anti–managed care movement that underlies them seem to have won the day. By 2001 Robinson announced "The End of Managed Care" in the *Journal of the American Medical Association*, asserting that care managers—cost-conscious employers, insurers who manage care, and physicians, unwilling managers of cost—are in full retreat. The consumer, Robinson claimed, had won. A similar theme was voiced by Havighurst in a 2002 article with a section titled "Managed Care Is Dead! Long Live Managed Care." Declines in enrollment data support the central thrust of these death claims, if not their extremity. Commercial enrollments in HMOs began to decline in 2000, and that trend continues as enrollments shifted to looser forms of managed care—preferred provider organizations and point-of-service plans—that are more popular with consumers. As of January 2009 managed care penetration was 50.3 percent of the US population (Managed Care On-Line 2009). At the same time, double-digit premium increases returned in 2001 for employer-sponsored health insurance, partially because costs were no longer being managed (Alliance for Health Reform 2002).[5] Premium increases continued to be high during the first decade of the twenty-first century, totaling 114 percent during the decade, far outpacing workers' earnings, which grew only 36 percent (Henry J. Kaiser Family Foundation 2012, 18).

Determinants of Regulatory Innovation

Most states had enacted their patient rights regulations by the end of 2000. A few states were finishing up in a few areas in 2001 and 2002, but by the end of 2002 patient rights were well established in the states. Thus, the legal stage of the managed care backlash seems to have ended. But it will surely go down in history as an unusually successful political and regulatory protest.

As in the last chapter, we are faced with a puzzle: The states took concerted action, this time against the managed care industry, while the federal government did not. And the states adopted their innovations between 1994 and 2001, a short diffusion period quite different from that of the state pharmacy assistance programs. Rather the adoptions of anti–managed care laws seem to be an example of what Graeme Boushey (2010) calls "a policy outbreak," a process characterized by rapid and sweeping policy change as compared with slow, incremental learning. He says that high-salience issues, which we argue described the shortcomings of managed care in the middle to late 1990s, are especially likely to produce a policy outbreak (Boushey 2010, 18). Also prone to policy outbreaks are issues of low complexity, which granted are not usually regulatory in nature, but in this case the issues are relatively simple. Also anti–managed care regulations fit the "high salience/low complexity" cell in Gormley's (1986) original typology. He argued that politicians are attracted by salience and repelled by complexity and that citizens' groups react the same way; business, conversely, likes low-salience issues. The pressure for accountability in this cell is intense, notes Gormley (1986, 606), which reinforces the motivation for quick legislative action.

Who was responsible for the protest against managed care? Interestingly, no definitive study of the protest has been conducted; ours is the first fifty-state analysis of the politics surrounding the adoption of anti–managed care legislation. Our analysis is informed by previous scholarship on the need to regulate managed care (e.g., Kinney 2002; Sorian and Feder 1999; Cauchi 1999; Robinson 2003), on the types of anti-HMO regulations (e.g., Noble and Brennan 1999; Miller 1997), and on the political and economic efficacy of anti–managed care regulation (Fox 1999; Stone 1999; Hall 2005; Hall and Agrawal 2003; Kronebusch, Schlesinger, and Thomas 2009).

Brown's (2001, 95) interviews from the second Community Tracking Study conducted in 1998–99 suggests that we focus on organized interests to understand why the backlash against managed care was successful. Interest organizations played a crucial role in states' adoption of managed care regulations, he argues.[6] Thus, the theoretical framework we adopted in other chapters, focusing on organized interest advocates, opponents, and the overall proportion of health interests, would seem to be appropriate for these regulatory innovations as well. Brown's interviews identified physicians as the only group in all twelve study sites that acted as the prime movers for adoption of anti–managed care regulations. These include measures that would ease physicians' own economic plight, which would address specialty physicians' agenda that patients enjoy direct access to their services, and also provide more patient-oriented rights.[7] The second source of demand for regulation Brown (2001, 96) identifies is the advocacy community—organizations representing patients with chronic diseases or disabilities, those concerned with the health of a particular demographic category, health reform groups, and economic and professional groups. The size of the advocacy community is quite variable. In liberal Massachusetts, for example, the coalition to reform managed care embraced ninety different organizations.

The key opponents of patient protection laws at the state level seem to have been the same ones who stopped it in Congress: business associations, managed care associations, and sometimes individual business firms and individual HMOs. The avoidance of regulation is an obvious incentive for HMOs and other managed care organizations. But their opposition may not have always been absolute or highly public. Brown (2001, 100; see also Sorian and Feder 1999) reported that instead of trying to kill regulations, managed care opponents often tried to work with legislators to produce reasonable regulations they could live with. Perhaps the most plausible interpretation is that when they saw the political handwriting on the wall, HMOs shifted to a stance designed to at least partially accommodate the inevitable. As for business interests, they opposed regulation as a blow against the cost-cutting effectiveness of managed care organizations, a fear that seems to have been confirmed by the upward trends in health costs reported above.

We added one more set of actors to this list of organized interest opponents—attorneys, who might prefer to manage managed care on a retail basis by use of malpractice suits rather than wholesale through regulatory activity. Finally, we also account for the size of the entire health interest system given Gray and Lowery's (1995a) finding that crowded interest systems make the passage of *any* legislation more difficult. Also in prior work Gray and Lowery (1997, 338) demonstrated that political action committee (PAC) sponsorship is part of an arms race among similar organized interests, all of which are seeking access to a common pool of elected officials. Thus, it is advantageous to measure and include PAC contributions from the health care industry in our model.

Although we find Brown's (2001) emphasis on the role of organized interests a congenial one, it is also incomplete to explain the adoption and stringency of a regulatory innovation. Another set of actors had a significant part in the drama—the politicians who adopted the laws mandating the regulatory requirements. Two hypotheses drawn from the internal determinants of innovation literature merit our attention. First, we have seen that public opinion turned sharply against managed care in the mid-1990s. Politicians are quite skilled in following public opinion (Erikson, Wright, and McIver 1993), and political scientists since V. O. Key (1949) have thought that the incentives to do so should be greater in states with more competitive political parties. Moreover, Gray and Lowery (1996) have argued that both opponents and supporters of the status quo tend to be more active in states with competitive parties. Thus, regulatory activity should be greater in states with more competitive political parties. Second, the anti–managed care movement was also identified as a consumer issue. Liberal states have generally been more predisposed to regulate on both economic and social issues (Eshbaugh-Soha and Meier 2008, 411). Therefore, states with more liberal electorates and greater Democratic control should have provided more fertile ground for supporters of managed care regulation.

Next, legislators might find that reliance on the wholesale regulatory solutions in their toolkits is more appealing in states with greater regulatory capacities. Thus, we predict that the states' capacities to regulate also played a role in the adoption and stringency of managed care reforms. We include an indicator of the administrative capacity of the states as well as the more general capacity measure of wealth.

And last, adoption of reforms is expected to be influenced by the severity of the problem or the need for the reform. One aspect of objective need for regulation is the extent to which a state's health care marketplace was dominated by managed care organizations. We will see that this varied markedly across the states. Support for regulation should have been stronger in states in which HMO penetration was extensive because consumers would have more opportunity for negative experiences and therefore lawmakers should hear more complaints. Another potential marker for objective need concerns the frequency of malpractice suits across the states. High relative numbers of such suits may provide a signal to elected officials that they have something to gain politically by attempting to regulate managed care, even if the lawsuits were not necessarily aimed at physicians employed by HMOs.[8]

External diffusion sources could not be incorporated into the model, for reasons that are explained below.

Testing the Hypotheses

In this section we describe the measures we will use to test the hypotheses laid out above and the nature of the research design used in this chapter.

Research Design

Before describing the measures, we should first note that both the unusually rapid pattern of adoptions and limits in data availability constrained how we were able to test the hypotheses. In terms of the latter, we could not secure reliable data about the year of adoption of three state regulations of HMOs. These included rules pertaining to internal grievance procedures, standing referrals, and access to obstetrician-gynecologist specialists. And where timing data are available on the other nine laws, it is clear that state regulations of HMOs diffused rapidly during the last part of the 1990s. Continuity of care provisions, for example, were adopted by twenty-one states, with all but one adoption falling between 1996 and 2002 and most falling between 1997 and 1999.[9] This pattern is repeated time and again; one or two states adopted a rule by 1995, 1996, or 1997. Within the next three years or so, other states followed, with adoptions fading rapidly after 1999, until only one or two took place in 2001 or 2002. This rapid diffusion makes it very difficult to analyze the data using a pooled design. The independent variables simply do not vary significantly over such a short period. Given missing data on the year of adoption of several regulations and the lack of variation on the independent variables, we chose to treat the data as a single cross section, with most of the independent variables measured by 1997 and 1999 average values.

Dependent Variables

The dependent variables are several versions of an index of intensity of state regulation of managed care organizations; they include the adoption of the innovation with the regulation's stringency. The several dependent variables are all constructed upon data on state adoption of regulations governing twelve kinds of activities by HMOs, as seen in table 4.1. The data sources for the dependent variables are listed in appendix table 4.1, and their descriptive statistics (means and standard deviations) are listed in appendix table 4.2. These rules and regulations are self- explanatory, given the descriptions in the table and our discussions above of the efforts of states to regulate managed care.[10] The simplest form of the dependent variable is a count of the number of these regulations states had adopted by 2002 (Chronbach's alpha = 0.63).[11] As seen in figure 4.1, only one state (North Carolina) adopted all twelve regulations, whereas two states (Wyoming and Mississippi) adopted only two.

Although these counts constitute the basis of all of our dependent variables, simple counts alone do not utilize the full range of information we have on these regulations. That is, several of the rules—liability laws or the right to sue, bans on provider financial incentives and gag rules, access to emergency rooms under a prudent layperson guideline, and use of ombudsman and report cards—are truly dichotomous in that states either have them or they do not. The stringency of the other six regulations varies, however, across the

Table 4.1 Types of Managed Care Regulations Adopted by the States

Highly restrictive regulations
1. Liability: Right to sue health plans for damages
2. Independent external review of appeals required Stringency varies by whether the external review is binding; those with binding reviews were coded 2, nonbinding reviews, 1.
3. Any willing provider law Stringency varies by breadth of coverage; laws limited to pharmacists were coded 1, laws applying to physicians, and most providers, were coded 3; others were coded 2.
4. Bans on provider financial incentives

Moderately restrictive regulations
5. Ombudsman program
6. Graduated levels of internal review Stringency varies by whether the HMO is required to assist in the filing for an internal review; laws coded 2 if yes and 1 if no. Stringency also varies by time frame for review; laws coded 2 if there is time frame and 1 if not.
7. Continuity of care protections Stringency varies by extent of coverage; laws coded 1 for 30 days coverage, 2 for 60, 3 for 90, 4 for 120, 5 for term pregnancy, 6 if until end of year, with 1 more point added if law covered medically necessary cases and pregnancies.
8. Standing referrals to specialists Stringency varies by extent of coverage; laws coded 0.5 if 6 months for dermatology only, 1 for standing referral for 1 year, 2 if specialists can coordinate care within scope of their practice, and 3 for no limit.
9. Direct access to obstetrician-gynecologists Stringency varies by extent of coverage; laws coded 1 if limited to 1 visit per year, 2 if no limits.

Less restrictive regulations
10. HMO report card established
11. Emergency room access under "prudent layperson" standard
12. Bans on gag rules

Source: Reprinted with permission from Gray, Lowery, and Godwin (2007a).

states. Regulations mandating independent external reviews of appeals, for example, are in some cases binding and in others not. In cases where stringency varies, we modified the simple count codes in the manner described in table 4.1. Again using independent external reviews as an example, states with nonbinding requirements were coded 1 and states with binding rules

Figure 4.1 Frequency Distribution of Anti–Managed Care Regulations Adopted by States

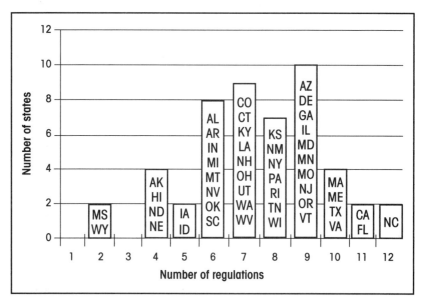

Source: Reprinted with permission from Gray, Lowery, and Godwin (2007b).

were assigned a code of 2. The second dependent variable, then, is the sum of the standardized scores for all twelve of the managed care regulations, with the coding of six of the rules expanded in order to account for variations in stringency.

The third and fourth versions of the dependent variable add another wrinkle to the analysis by ranking the twelve regulations by substantive importance rather than treating all regulations as if they were equally burdensome to the managed care industry. We address this variation by weighing the twelve regulations on a 3-point scale tapping the importance of the regulation.[12] As seen in table 4.1, three regulations—those concerning HMO report cards, emergency room access under a prudent layperson standard, and bans on gag rules—were assigned a score of 1, indicating that we consider these to be the least restrictive of the regulations. Report cards are the type of information that health plans actually like to make available—data that allow consumers to compare competing plans on quality, finances, and service. The ban on gag clauses in physician contracts is of lesser impact because no health plan actually had such a clause (General Accounting Office 1997) and because organizations have other ways to motivate physicians. And though the "prudent layperson" standard for emergency room admission may cost health plans money, it is hard to argue against the idea, especially since 1997, when Medicaid began to require it.

In the top category, assigned a value of 3, are four laws that are perceived to really tie HMO management's hands in dealing with providers or patients: being sued by patients, facing binding external review, not being able to incentivize providers, and having to accept "any willing quack" in the parlance of the industry. With such laws in place, HMO managers fear the costs of malpractice and external review claims and bad publicity from lawsuits. If HMOs have to accept just any physician, they may have less ability to guarantee a desired level of quality of care (or cost).

In the middle tier, assigned a value of 2, are policies that modify the behavior of managed care organizations in some way but do not threaten their very survival. The requirements for internal review, continuity of care after the physician or the patient (if terminally ill or pregnant) leaves the plan, standing referral to a specialist (without going through a gatekeeper each time), and direct access to obstetrician-gynecologists (without going through a gatekeeper) are not anathemas as concepts. HMOs' opposition depends more on their stringency and their implementation—how long is continuity of care required, and under what circumstances. The ombudsman program is also placed in the middle tier because opposition to it depends more upon the scope and resources of the office than on its existence. These importance values were then multiplied by either the simple counts of the first dependent variable or the standardized stringency values of the second dependent variable to generate *weighted* versions of each. Although the four dependent variables represent distinct efforts to account for variations in the stringency and/or the substantive importance of the twelve regulations, they are all closely related to each other. The weakest correlation among the four measures is +.90.[13]

Measures of the Independent Variables

The mean and standard deviations of all of the independent variables are reported in the appendix in table A4.2, whereas the sources of those variables are reported in table A4.3.[14]

VARIABLE SET ONE: ORGANIZED INTERESTS

The first set of independent variables addresses our core concerns about organized interests. We employ several variables tapping the relative presence of organized interests that might influence the rate of adoption of anti-HMO regulations. All are based on state lobby registration data collected by Gray and Lowery and recoded by Gray and colleagues (2005b). Not all health interest organizations are concerned about the regulation of HMOs. Still, we examined a number of different coding schemes for eighteen finer categories of substantive health interests in the data.[15] These included both broad and narrow definitions of allies and enemies of regulation, as well as including these in models separately and as ratios. In many cases, for reasons that are discussed below, these generated only very weak results. In the end we adopted for inclusion in our estimating models only four measures of the relative presence of specific kinds of health interests within state interest systems—those tapping the specific kinds of interests noted by Brown (2001) based on his interviews from the second Community Tracking Study in 1998–99. Two of the measures indicate the relative presence within health interest communities of two subguilds that would be expected to *favor* HMO regulation: health advocacy organizations (citizens' groups promoting consumers' interests) and independent medical care providers (independent clinics and medical groups and individual practices). These represent the interests of citizens and independent medical providers, respectively. The relative presence of each is measured by the average of their 1997 and 1999 proportions of all health interest organizations.

Two types of health interest organizations were expected to *oppose* HMO regulation. The first are individual HMOs and the trade organizations representing them. Although we expect the HMO coefficient to be negative, as noted above, some scholars pointed out that in the end organizations representing HMOs did not take a confrontational stance against regulation, but rather a more accommodative position in working with lawmakers. We use a two-tailed test in order to test for both possibilities. A second set of health interest organizations that are expected to oppose regulation are health business interests, including employer health plans, employer health coalitions, and insurance companies. Employer health coalitions tend to be protective of HMOs because of their cost-effectiveness in providing employee medical care and because they were fearful of regulations that might add costs to the employer.

We also include two other measures of the structure of the interest community that might plausibly influence HMO regulation, both of which are measured by their average proportion of the *entire* interest community in a state in 1997 and 1999 rather than of the health guild per se. The first measures the relative number of interest registrations by organizations representing lawyers, who might well prefer minimal regulation so as to protect a lucrative business in defending consumers through retail, case-by-case use of malpractice suits.

And to tap the gridlock, noted by Gray and Lowery (1995b) within crowded interest communities, the estimating models include the average of the 1997 and 1999 proportions of state interest communities made up of health interest organizations.[16] Both these variables should depress regulatory activity.

We have, then, six measures of the structure of the interest communities that are expected to influence levels of regulatory activity. Such activity should be suppressed when there is relatively greater representation by health business, HMO, and lawyer interests, as well as when interest systems are crowded. Greater relative representation by health advocacy and independent medical care interests should promote greater regulatory activity. Somewhat surprisingly, given that the measures are proportions, they are only weakly related to each other.[17] In part this is a function of the fact that health interest communities comprise more than advocacy, business, independent care providers, and HMO interests; together, their average proportions of the health interest communities during 1997 and 1999 sum to only 25.65 percent. More substantively important, however, the weak correlations among these variables suggest that we are not seeing a simple pattern of mobilization and counter-mobilization whereby proposed legislation simply brings to the table more registrants of all types (Gray et al. 2005b). To foreshadow an important part of our findings, for example, the correlation (–0.09) between the average of the 1997 and 1999 proportions of HMOs and independent care provider registrations is especially weak and incorrectly signed.

The campaign finance data from the National Institute on Money in Politics do not go back very far in time, and thus we were not able to include a PAC contribution measure in our time series models in other chapters. However, the use of a cross-sectional design in this chapter allows us to include in the model financial contributions from health organizations to state-level political campaigns. The specific measure is the proportion of all PAC contribution dollars in the state coming from the health sector. All nonparty, nonindividual contributions to state candidates made by organizations in the six health categories coded by the institute were included, as well as organizations with health-related names that we selected from three additional categories. Data are from 1998 unless the state did not hold an election that year; in those cases data from the next available year with state legislative elections were substituted.

VARIABLE SET TWO: POLITICAL VARIABLES

Three measures of the ideological and partisan makeup of a state are included in our model specification. The first is party competition, measured by the average of folded Ranney indices for 1997 and 1999.[18] Low values indicate one-party dominance, and high values convey high levels of party competition. The second political measure is the average of the 1997 and 1999 values of Erikson, Wright, and McIver's (1993) indicator of public opinion liberalism. This measure is widely used in the political science literature and has been employed in health policy research as well (Kousser 2002; Miller 2006). The final political measures are the averages of 1997 and 1999 values of Democratic Party control of state legislatures and of Democratic governorships. States were coded 1 if Democrats controlled a legislative chamber and 1 if they controlled the governorship, with Republican control coded 0.[19] More regulatory activity is expected in states with high levels of party competition, states with more liberal electorates, and states with higher levels of Democratic Party control of either the state legislature or the governor's office.[20]

VARIABLE SET THREE: REGULATORY CAPACITY

We use two measures of the states' regulatory capacity. The first is a measure of the states' administrative capacity in 1999 developed by the Government Performance Project, a study conducted by the Maxwell School of Citizenship and Public Affairs at Syracuse University and *Governing* magazine (Barrett and Greene 1999). States were graded on their management capacity in financial, capital, and human resources and their practices promoting managing for results and use of information technology. The "grades" were averaged to produce an overall grade ranging from A to F. We then recoded these final grades to a score running from a value of five for outstanding capacity to a value of one for a failing grade. Alabama had the lowest score of 1.5, whereas Missouri, Virginia, Utah, and Washington were judged to have the strongest administrative capacity, with scores of 4.2. Our second measure of administrative capacity assumes that wealthier states can afford to invest more in their bureaucracies than can poorer states (see Eshbaugh-Soha and Meier 2008). We measure state economic wealth by the average of 1997 and 1999 per capita gross state product.

VARIABLE SET FOUR: PROBLEM SEVERITY/NEED VARIABLES

We employ two measures of the states' need for HMO regulation. The first captures HMO penetration of a state's health market, as measured by the average of the 1997 and 1999 proportions of a state's population enrolled in HMOs. The second measure taps the rate of successful malpractice suits in the states. Ideally, we would employ some indicator of the rate of successful suits against HMOs in the period just before the adoption of the several regula-

Figure 4.2 Number of Newspaper Stories on Managed Care Reform, 1994–2003

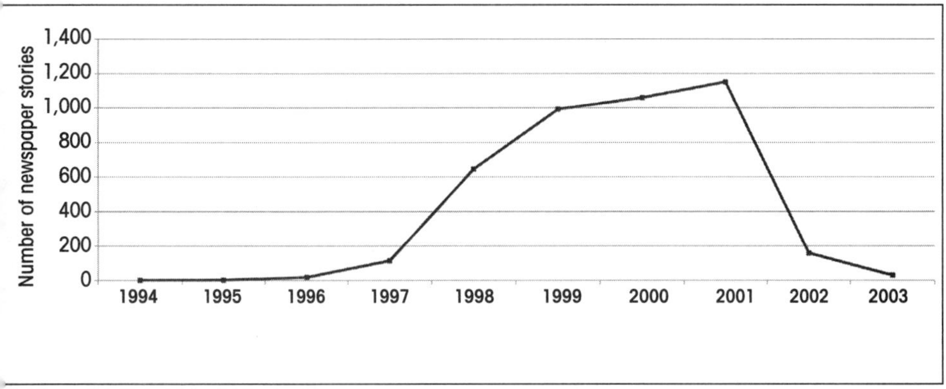

Source: Lexis/Nexis, calculated by the authors.

tions. But such data were not available. As a surrogate, we employ the number of malpractice payments (successful suits or settlements) per 1,000 medical practitioners in a state from September 1990 through 1996. Although less than ideal, this measure demonstrates considerable variation across the states: Alabama had a low of only 6.87 payments, whereas Michigan had a high of 44.46 per 1,000 practitioners. This measure assumes that the variation observed from 1990 through 1996 continued to characterize the states during the late 1990s. This is not an unreasonable assumption, given that this was precisely the time when public opinion turned against managed care. We expect that regulatory activity will be greater in states with higher rates of successful suits and higher levels of HMO penetration.[21]

OMITTED VARIABLES: REGIONAL AND NATIONAL DIFFUSION

Due to the cross-sectional research design employed in this chapter, we are not able to include in the model either the interstate or national diffusion measures that are used in other chapters. However, the fact that anti–managed care legislation spread so rapidly throughout the states in the late 1990s suggests that diffusion or contagion might have been at work in the adoption of this reform. Figure 4.2 graphs national attention paid to anti–managed care activities, using an annual count of the terms "patients' bill of rights," "managed care reform," or "HMO regulations" found in newspaper headlines or

Table 4.2 Ordinary-Least-Squares Model of Determinants of HMO Regulation by States, Cross-Sectional Model Using 1997–1999 Averages, $n = 50$

	Unweighted		Weighted	
	No. of Provisions	Stringency of Provisions	No. of Provisions	Stringency of Provisions
Interest organization variables				
Health advocacy proportion	.03	.05	.08	.10
	(0.58)	(0.41)	(0.59)	(0.33)
Independent care provider proportion	.02***	.04***	.03***	.07***
	(3.28)	(3.20)	(2.97)	(2.77)
HMO proportion	.17+	.39+	.38+	.86+
	(1.87)	(1.84)	(1.82)	(1.86)
Health business proportion	−.09	−.15	−.20	−.38
	(−0.81)	(−0.70)	(−0.90)	(−0.78)
Health proportion of all registrations	−.10**	−.19**	−.22***	−.46**
	(−2.46)	(−2.23)	(−2.46)	(−2.29)
Law proportion of all registrations	−.52*	−.94	−1.26*	−2.31*
	(−1.58)	(−1.26)	(−1.61)	(−1.34)
PAC variables				
Health proportion of all contributions	−7.92*	−32.05**	−13.44	−61.59**
	(−1.33)	(−2.38)	(−0.96)	(−2.00)
Political variables				
Opinion liberalism	2.99	5.90	6.41	13.20
	(1.00)	(0.87)	(0.91)	(0.84)
Folded Ranney index	7.68***	20.33***	15.20**	43.03***
	(2.65)	(3.09)	(2.21)	(2.84)
Democratic governor	−.46	.18	−1.03	1.26
	(−0.79)	(0.14)	(−0.75)	(0.42)
Democratic legislature	1.30**	2.69**	2.80**	6.24**
	(2.13)	(1.95)	(1.94)	(1.96)
Capacity variables				
Administrative capacity	1.01**	1.99**	1.97**	3.50*
	(2.31)	(2.00)	(1.91)	(1.53)
Per capita GSP	−78.75	−35.16	−148.66	−59.24
	(−1.35)	(−0.27)	(−1.07)	(−0.19)
Need variables				
HMO penetration	0.05**	.07*	.07*	.08
	(2.05)	(1.37)	(1.33)	(0.67)
Malpractice suit rate	−.03	−.06	−.04	−.07
	(−0.82)	(−0.78)	(−0.48)	(−0.36)
Constant	.79	−20.67**	2.53	−40.91**
	(0.20)	(−2.34)	(0.27)	(−2.01)
R^2	.69	.70	.60	.63

Note: t statistics in parentheses.
* $p < 0.10$, ** $p < 0.05$, *** $p < 0.01$, one-tailed test; + $p < 0.10$, ++ $p < 0.05$, +++ $p < 0.01$, two-tailed test.
Source: Calculated by the authors.

lead paragraphs by Lexis/Nexis. The graph shows national attention peaking between 1999 and 2001, whereas state passage had topped out in 1997; as a result the correlation of the trend in attention with the passage of state regulations is a modest +.235. It seems likely that the attention graph is picking up stories surrounding consideration of patient protection by the US Congress, which took place in 2001 after the time when most states had already acted to rein in managed care organizations.

Findings

The ordinary-least-squares results for the four variations of our dependent variable are presented in table 4.2. All the models generated strong coefficients of determination. Given the high correlations among the four dependent variables, it is not surprising that the four models generate largely similar results. We therefore discuss the estimates and their interpretation in blocks running across all four models. First, what is the influence of *interest organizations*? As noted above, our search for evidence indicating interest influence on states' regulatory activity extended far beyond the specific measures listed in table 4.2. We examined numerous configurations of interest organization variables in our search for significant effects. These largely generated null results. However, one consistent effect observed across all models in table 4.2 concerns the gridlock hypothesis, as indicated by the consistently negative and highly significant estimates for health organizations' registrations as a proportion of all registrations (three at the 0.05 level and one at the 0.01 level). The results indicate that having an interest system made up of a greater percentage of health lobby registrants depresses regulatory activity across the board: The higher the proportion of health lobbying organizations, the fewer HMO regulations adopted and the weaker the stringency of those regulations. These results had meaningful substantive impact. For example, using predictions from the model of unweighted total provisions, the states with the minimum proportion of health lobbying organizations will have twelve provisions, compared with only five laws for states with the maximum proportion of health lobbying organizations.

The second consistent effect observed among the interest group variables in table 4.2 is that all the independent care provider estimates are positively signed, as predicted, and highly significant at the 0.01 level. When relatively more independent providers lobby, state legislatures respond by enacting more regulations on managed care, and they make those laws more stringent. Brown (2001) seems to have been right about provider dominance. And again the results yield substantive importance. Using predictions from the model of unweighted total provisions, the states at the minimum for the independent provider lobby will have three provisions, compared with twelve for states with the maximum proportion of independent provider lobbying organizations.

Another way in which organized interests fairly consistently exercised influence over anti–managed care regulations was through using political action committees to make financial contributions to electoral campaigns. In states where health PACs' contributions constituted a higher proportion of total PAC donations, regulatory activity tended to be depressed as compared with states in which the health sector's largesse was a lower proportion of all campaign funds. The effect was weakly negative on the adoption of such regulations ($p = 0.10$ for the number of provisions adopted and not significant for their weighted number), but solidly significant at the 0.05 level for the stringency of such provisions for either the weighted or unweighted versions. Where relatively more campaign money originates from the health sector, the stringency or content of the regulations is watered down as compared with those states in which the health care industry's money is relatively less. Again, as we saw for the pharmaceutical assistance programs, organized interests often have more influence behind the scenes in the nitty-gritty of the legislation than on whether or not a law is passed.

Beyond these effects, evidence of interest group influence is either weak or mixed. The coefficients on the law organization variables are consistently negative, as predicted for opponents of regulation, and three of four coefficients are modestly significant at the 0.10 level. Thus, it appears that the legal profession would have preferred the status quo in which managed care's patients had to rely on them to sue corporations rather than to see consumer complaints taken care of by regulation. The other opponent of regulation— health business interests—also generated the expected negative coefficients, but none were significant. Apparently, they did little by themselves to stem the tide of anti–managed care regulations.

As expected, the health advocacy estimates are consistently positive, yet none are significant. The weak results for advocacy groups are especially surprising given the strong expectations of Brown (2001) based on twelve case studies of regulatory reform. One possibility is that the influence of citizens' groups is lost in the glare of the political variables. That is, liberal and Democratic politicians might well be expected to be attentive to such organizations so that the influence of the former is expressed *through* the presence of the latter. However, the advocacy coefficients remain small even when the three political variables are dropped, whereas all else remains as reported in table 4.2.

In contrast, all four estimates for the HMO proportion of all interest organizations variable are incorrectly signed, and using a two-tailed test, the relationships are weakly significant at the 0.10 level. This indicates that a greater relative presence of HMOs, who are expected to oppose regulation of their own industry, actually promoted greater regulation and, even more surprisingly, greater stringency. Perhaps it was the case, as some have suggested (Brown 2001; Sorian and Feder 1999), that HMO organizations jumped on the reform bandwagon when they saw such regulations were going to pass. Obviously, this is a puzzle to which we must return in the conclusion of the chapter. For now, however, it is worth noting that this counterintuitive positive relationship helps to explain the failure of HMOs' friends in killing regulatory reform. At least in terms of any kind of consistent effect associated with relative numbers of lobby registrations, there do not seem to have been many strongly effective opponents of reform.

Strong results were generated for two of four *political* variables. All four of the party competition estimates were positively signed, as expected, and significantly different from 0 at the 0.01 level in three cases and at the 0.05 level in one case. These results indicate that regulatory activity was greater in states with more competitive party systems. And all four of the Democratic Party legislative control estimates were positive and significant, all at the 0.05 level. This means that legislatures under Democratic Party control adopted more regulations of all types, more stringent regulations, and substantively more important regulations. However, whether a state had a Democratic governor had no discernible effect upon its likelihood of pursuing regulatory reform of managed care. The explanation for this finding is likely to be found in scholars' views that legislatures, at both the federal and state levels, are usually the more dominant players in the regulatory process than are chief executives (Teske 2004, chap. 13; Meier and Garman 1995). Moreover, Teske (2004) argues that the legislature's impact can be captured by a simple dichotomous variable, whereas the governor's influence is harder to measure.

Although the opinion liberalism estimates are correctly signed to suggest that more liberal states had higher levels of regulatory activity, they generated statistically insignificant estimates. Evidently, public opinion liberalism works through the political variables of party competition and Democratic legislative control, both of which clearly heightened the levels of anti-HMO regulatory activity.

Positive results were also generated for one of the *capacity* variables, the one that specifically measured administrative capacity. We hypothesized that states would be more likely to regulate if they had a stronger capacity to do so. The estimates of administrative capacity generated the expected positive estimates.

Administrative capacity was significant at the 0.05 level three times and at the 0.10 level for the weighted stringency measure. However, the more general measure of state capacity—economic wealth as measured by per capita gross state product—was incorrectly signed and not significant. It is possible that anti-HMO regulations consume relatively few financial resources but rather are an administrative burden to implement. As such, state wealth is less of a factor than with other kinds of regulations, for example, environmental protection. Still, it seems that states with strong administrative systems were more likely to regulate HMOs.

Mixed results were generated for the *problem severity or policy need* variables measuring HMO penetration and the rate of malpractice suits. HMO penetration was positively related to anti–managed care regulatory activity. The coefficient for the number of provisions adopted was positive and significant at the 0.05 level, though the stringency coefficient and the weighted number of provisions coefficient were only modestly significant at the 0.10 level, with the other coefficient lacking significance. It seems, then, in states where HMOs have a relatively greater presence, more regulations against them are likely to be enacted and are somewhat more likely to be substantively important and to be stringent. This pattern implies that HMO penetration is at least a latent indicator of problem severity. The second measure of policy need—the malpractice suit rate—is incorrectly signed and not significant across all four models. The rush to regulate HMOs therefore seems to be related to their penetration of health markets, not to the rate of malpractice suits/settlements.[22] The lack of a finding for the latter variable may be due to the fact that it is a proxy variable, including all reported settlements rather than only settlements against HMOs.

Conclusion

If politics, both electoral and interest group, largely determined how active states were in regulating managed care organizations during the late 1990s, how are we to understand that politics? Our organized interest results are generally quite consistent across the several measures of regulatory activity: The more health care organizations registered to lobby, proportionately, the fewer regulations enacted and the less stringent are those that do pass. Similarly, where health PACs contribute more money proportionately, the stringency of regulations is reduced. The strongest advocacy lobby turned out to be the independent medical care providers; they had a clear positive impact on both the number of anti–managed care regulations passed and the teeth in those regulations. However, the finding that greater representation by HMOs in the health lobbying community would also lead to greater regulatory activity leaves us with an interesting puzzle.

At least three explanations might be invoked to explain this surprising finding. It does not seem that the surprising positive estimates for HMO registrations are a function of mobilization and counter-mobilization, whereby prospective legislation brought out more lobbying organizations of all stripes. If this were true, then the positive estimates for HMO registrants would be evidence of extensive—if unsuccessful—opposition to state regulation. We have seen above, however, that greater relative representation by independent care providers is not associated with greater relative HMO representation (–0.09). Accordingly, it does not seem that we can account for the puzzlingly positive HMO estimates in this manner.

A second explanation would invoke Stigler's (1971) and Peltzman's (1976) assertion that regulation is usually provided at the behest of those who are regulated. That is, the positive estimates for HMO representation may really reflect the efforts of allies rather than of enemies of reform. We do not find this explanation plausible for two reasons. First, if this explanation were valid, it would only shift the locus of our puzzle from the HMO coefficients to the estimates for the independent provider organizations. That is, if regulatory "reforms" were actually supportive of HMOs from the start, why did the independent provider variable generate *positive* and highly significant estimates? Why would independent physicians have supported regulation that was merely symbolic and "toothless"? Second and more important, we have seen little evidence to suggest that HMOs looked favorably upon regulations of the type included in our dependent variables. A look at the website of American Association of Health Plans (AAHP), managed care's trade organization, shows just the opposite. There one could find a report on "Health Plan Liability: What You Need to Know" (AAHP 2001). The thrust of the report was that expanded health plan liability would diminish the quality of medical care and add substantially to health care costs. Or one could read a summary of a study on why health care costs have risen; it attributed half the increase in costs to government regulation, runaway litigation, and increased bargaining power resulting from provider consolidations (AAHP 2002). Managed care's official position appeared to be squarely against the regulations we are studying.

A third candidate explanation of our puzzling findings is that HMOs, facing a tsunami of political pressure in support of regulation and having a host of other—often more important—issues on the health policy agenda, opted to go along with reform, perhaps participating in the lawmaking process so as to diminish its negative consequences for their businesses. This explanation has a little more resonance, in that Brown and Eagan (2004) noted instances in California and Massachusetts when HMOs were motivated to bargain constructively over regulations because they were fighting off more frightening ballot initiatives at the time. Moreover, when HMOs do choose to negotiate behind closed doors, they often find state lawmakers ready to deal; lawmakers do not want to kill the goose that brought cost savings to the state employees' health plan or to many corporations' health plans. This explanation has some merit, especially if HMOs were being strategic at the last minute. Also recall that HMOs were dealing with a high-salience situation, in which business inherently has less of an advantage than on low-salience issues. In some states negotiating might have been the best tactic an HMO could adopt.

Even if we could solve the specific puzzle over interpreting the HMO finding, our other results also have interesting implications. We found a strong role for party politics as measured by party competition and Democratic Party legislative, but not gubernatorial, control in enhancing the amount and stringency of anti–managed care regulation. These results leave us with another conundrum: Simply put, does this strong role for politics represent public officials' political pandering to public opinion and/or interest organizations? Or is this a case of democratic responsiveness? Obviously, our results cannot really answer this question. Indeed, political pandering to one person may well constitute democratic responsiveness to another. But it is still an interesting question, for which the best evidence is the rapid diffusion of HMO regulations during the late 1990s, accompanied by the equally rapid diffusion of its more symbolic cousin—the "patients' bill of rights." The rapid spread of adoptions resembles more the kind of democratic frenzy, policy outbreak, or bandwagon effect associated with the rapid diffusion of tax cut proposals during the era of the tax revolt (Sigelman, Lowery, and Smith 1983; Mahoney 2003) than with normal politics observed even on other kinds of health policy issues, such as pharmacy assistance programs. This at least raises the possibility of political pandering. That is, HMOs were once very popular, but the backlash against their strictness may have been a bandwagon upon which many politicians decided to leap for relatively little policy purpose.

However, other evidence suggests that the politics of anti–managed care laws was normal, albeit accomplished in short order. We found some of the predicted relationships in our data for the state capacity and problem severity measures. States with greater administrative capacity were more likely to pass laws regulating managed care. Likewise for the policy need variable of HMO penetration; states with relatively more HMOs tended to adopt more regulations. These patterns were associated with more typical regulatory processes. Finally, a recent study by Kronebusch, Schlesinger, and Thomas (2009) based upon a survey of physicians concludes that the managed care regulations adopted in the 1990s were strikingly effective. Despite ERISA and limitations on states' enforcement ability, these regulations had an impact on health plan behavior and on medical practice: "It challenges those critics who had dismissed managed care reform as impractical given those limitations" (Kronebusch, Schlesinger, and Thomas 2009, 254). Their findings that regulations are effective are not consistent with the political pandering thesis, but rather with the normal politics thesis. Overall, we believe that the passage of anti-HMO regulations in the 1990s is best explained by the same set of variables that explain other health reforms that diffused over longer periods.

As the era of HMO regulation ended, its critics proclaimed that managed care was dead; indeed, its enrollment peaked in 1999–2000 and has since declined. But many patients were shifted to preferred provider organizations so that managed care enrollment still totaled 126.4 million in 2009, with slightly more than half that number in HMOs (Managed Care On-Line 2009). Generally speaking, today's HMOs have "loosened up" in comparison with those in the 1990s in order to meet the demands of their customers whose memories appear to be very short. In the 2009 congressional debate over health care reform, private-sector health cooperatives were proposed (see Sack 2009a) without anyone pointing out that these sounded a lot like the early HMOs. Indeed, the ones held up as models, such as the Group Health Cooperative of Puget Sound founded in 1947, *were* the early HMOs. In the end, no type of "public option" was included in the final bill. Instead the Patient Protection and Affordable Care Act of 2010 authorized "new ideas" such as "accountable care organizations" to replace fee-for-service providers, "patient-centered medical homes" that would integrate all care for patients, and rely on capitated payments (Durenberger 2010; Weil and Scheppach 2010). All these carry familiar undertones of HMOs or "déjà vu all over again," as former US senator and HMO champion David Durenberger (R) put it (2010). Thus, it appears that HMOs will be part of our future, and perhaps may even be embraced once again by the left and the right alike.

Notes

1. Minnesota's Paul Ellwood convinced President Nixon of the merits of the idea, based upon the savings achieved in the Twin Cities marketplace by Group Health and other HMOs; Ellwood also coined the term "HMO."

2. An exception to this exclusive pattern of activity during the 1990s is the adoption of laws requiring "Report Cards" for HMOs. Minnesota first required them in 1974; no more states adopted the idea until 1994.

3. The National Committee on Quality Assurance, which is the national accrediting body for HMOs, had already made external review of medical necessity denials a requirement for accreditation in July 2000.

4. The *Aetna* decision in 2004 ran the other way because the Court ruled that the state of Texas cannot create new substantive rights; i.e., it cannot force an HMO to provide any specific set of benefits. This doctrine is not contrary to the Court's previous ruling in *Rush Prudential* or *Kentucky Association*, according to Sebok (2004).

5. Havighurst (2002) predicted this rise in health care costs after the regulatory backlash compelled managed care to loosen up, a trend that may bring back tight cost controls.

6. See also Ross (1999), who applies Alford's model of structural interests to the regulation of behavioral health care, classifying mental health providers in organized professional guilds as dominant structural interests, managed care organizations as challenging structural interests, and patient and consumer groups as repressed structural interests.

7. In the third wave of the Community Tracking Study (1998–2000), Brown and Eagan (2004) expected to find physicians reempowered by virtue of their triumph over managed care. However, after a study of four policies at twelve sites, they report that providers wield power only when they are united among themselves, when they ally with other interests, and when they face little or no opposition (Brown and Eagan 2004, 1062). Physicians have not yet regained sovereignty, they concluded.

8. Malpractice payment reports must be submitted to the National Practitioner Data Bank when an insurance company or self-insured entity (but not a self-insured individual) makes a payment for the benefit of a licensed health care practitioner in satisfaction of a malpractice claim. A state's malpractice rate may be underreported if a physician is allowed to hide behind the "corporate shield" of the codefendant HMO. If the practitioner is named in the claim but not in the settlement, no report has to be filed in the Data Bank.

9. In one of a handful of oddities, Minnesota mandated use of an ombudsman in 1974 while no other state adopted such requirements until 1995. In the end, we treat Minnesota as part of the general cross section with independent variables coded in the late 1990s in order to preserve degrees of freedom. In effect, for whatever reason Minnesota adopted this rule in 1974, our model expects that it would have adopted it in the late 1990s had it not done so earlier.

10. Our selection of laws regulating managed care was guided principally by

the study "Tracking State Oversight of Managed Care" (Milbank Memorial Fund and Reforming States Group (1999). The Milbank Memorial Fund is a national foundation that studies health policy. The Reforming States Group is an association of health policy leaders from the legislative and executive branches of the states, making them uniquely qualified to select important policies. From their list of five policies affecting consumers, we selected four: the right to sue health plans for damages (liability), the requirement for independent external review of appeals, the requirement for a graduated internal review of appeals (all states require some internal grievance process), and an ombudsman program. This source had a second list of ten policies affecting the patient–provider relationship (i.e., these policies would be of more interest to physicians and other providers). But several of these are of interest to patients, too. From their list of ten we selected seven: any-willing-provider laws, bans on provider financial incentives, continuity of care protections, standing referrals to specialists, direct access to obstetrician-gynecologists, emergency room access under the "prudent layperson" standard, and bans on "gag" rules. Policies not selected were due to data unavailability. We then canvassed the websites of the Kaiser Family Foundation, the NCSL, and the Health Policy Tracking Service to find dates of adoption, the stringency of the regulations, and other policies we might have overlooked. Through this process, we became aware of report cards rules and added these to the consumer protection set. Scaling analysis indicated that there was no reason to treat the two sets separately. They were combined in a single index of regulatory activity. Importantly, we did not measure whether states adopted a "Patient Bill of Rights." All but four states had adopted such measures by 2002. Indeed, several states adopted such laws several times! Closer inspection, however, suggests that these laws were a mixture of apples and oranges whose primary value resided in their politically appealing label. We focus instead on the specific regulations states adopted that had substantive meaning for the ways in which HMOs operate and/ or interact with patients.

11. Although our basic dependent variables *count* numbers of regulations, we do not think that it is appropriate to treat this measure as a "count" variable for the simple reason that its components are not recurring events. Once a state mandates use of an ombudsman program, it need not do so again. Still, the ordinary-least-squares regression analysis of the model using the simple "count" variable was also estimated using Poisson and negative binomial estimation procedures. The substantive results of these models were essentially identical to those reported in table 4.2.

12. To some extent, our classification of the importance of the regulations reflects how they were discussed in the health policy literature and the general press during the late 1990s. Even more important, one of the authors served on the consumer board of directors of a large HMO for nine years and was chair for two years. Thus, our coding of importance reflects to a considerable degree how the HMO industry evaluated the threat of the proposed regulations on the conduct of business.

13. The correlation between the simple count measure and the other three

measures is as follows: the standardized stringency measure (0.94), the weighted count measure (0.98), and the weighted standardized stringency measure (0.92). The correlation of the standardized stringency measure with the weight count variable is 0.90 and with the weighted standardized stringency measures 0.97. The correlation of the two weighted measures is 0.93.

14. Given the choice to utilize a cross-sectional model with fifteen predictor variables, several tests were conducted for all four models. White's test and the Breusch-Pagan-Godfrey test indicate no evidence of heteroscedasticity. Additionally, with a mean variance inflation factor of 1.72, there is no evidence of multicollinearity.

15. For a more complete description of these coding categories, see Gray et al. (2005b). Only thirty-one organizations in the 1999 health population could not be so coded. The largest health subguilds, constituting half of all health registrations, were seven categories providing direct patient care.

16. To some extent, the proportional measure of the size of the health guild taps relative rather than absolute numbers, which is the true focus of the gridlock hypothesis. Still, the model also includes gross state product, which is strongly related to the number of lobbying organizations found in the states (Gray and Lowery 1996). This should partially control for absolute size and allow our proportional or relative measure to tap the gridlock effect.

17. The proportion of the health interest community composed of advocacy organizations is negatively correlated with all three other proportions: HMOs (–0.26), independent care provider organizations (–0.10), and health business organizations (–0.32). The correlations of the proportion of independent care provider registrants with HMO (–0.09) and health business interest registrants (0.26) are similarly small as is the correlation between the proportions of the health interest system composed of health business interests and HMOs (0.22).

18. The fifty-state average was used for Nebraska, which has missing values on the Ranney index due to its nonpartisan, single chamber legislature, in order to preserve degrees of freedom. The results do not change markedly, however, when Nebraska is dropped from the analysis.

19. The few cases of split party control were coded 0.50.

20. Somewhat surprisingly, the three measures are only weakly correlated with each other. The Ranney index is correlated at only the –0.01 level with opinion liberalism and 0.12 with Democratic Party control. The opinion liberalism and Democratic Party control measures generated a correlation coefficient of only 0.21.

21. The two measures, however, are only weakly and negatively correlated with each other (–0.16).

22. We also examined a range of interactions among the policy need and political variables to little effect.

CHAPTER 5

Universal Health Care in the States

During the 1990s the states and the federal government addressed many of the same health care issues—universal coverage, regulation of managed care, and prescription drug coverage for seniors. But, as we have seen, the outcome was often different, with health reforms being enacted later or not at all at the federal level. In chapter 3 we saw that by 2004, thirty-four states had passed some kind of pharmaceutical assistance law, using state funds to pay for a portion of the cost of drugs for eligible senior residents. In chapter 4 we learned that between 1994 and 2001, the fifty states passed more than nine hundred different laws regulating managed care. But in this chapter we examine a diffusion process with a different policy outcome. Despite a number of incremental policy events—studies, bill introductions, the passage of laws by one or both legislative chambers, and sometimes the signing of these bills into law—the states collectively have not been successful in achieving universal health care coverage for their citizens.

At the national level, however, on March 23, 2010, when President Barack Obama signed the Patient Protection and Affordable Care Act (ACA), the nation took a major step toward (near) universal care. But even this comprehensive legislation did not contain a "public option," that is, a publicly sponsored health plan that would compete with private insurers to drive down premiums and ultimately health care costs. Such an option was first proposed in California (Halpin and Harbage 2010), was picked up by presidential candidate John Edwards during the 2008 campaign, and was ultimately endorsed by candidates Hillary Clinton and Barack Obama. The public option was included in the House of Representatives bill, but not in the Senate bill due to Senator Joe Lieberman's filibuster threat as well as the opposition of the Republican Party and its interest group allies. However, the public option could still be reborn at the state level, where a state may offer such an option through its new insurance exchange; indeed, that is just what the state of Vermont did in 2011 when it enacted Green Mountain Care, a single-payer plan. Thus, the analyses in this chapter may help serve as a road map for understanding states' actions in the future as they develop their insurance exchanges.

We are interested in the states' failures as well as their policy successes for several reasons. First, we want to know if the same forces credited with impeding national health care reform for so long have also limited state efforts to secure universal coverage. As explained in chapter 1, at the national level, organized interests are often credited with stymieing broad-based reform of the health care system.[1] Have the same organized interests also blocked universal health insurance legislation in the states? Second, why have the states been so successful in regulating managed care organizations and adopting pharmaceutical assistance programs, but less so in enacting and sustaining universal coverage? Examining the determinants of policy activity on universal coverage enables us to compare these results with our similar studies on more successful health care policies in chapters 3 and 4. We return to this question in the book's final chapter. Third and more broadly, we are interested in the prospects of incremental policy reform versus policy punctuations. That is, the states have hardly been inactive in trying to expand access to health insurance. Studies have been commissioned and bills have been considered and sometimes passed into law, even if less often implemented. Did these incremental steps take us anywhere? Berkman and Reenock (2004) assert that policy activity in the past can make full-fledged reform more likely in the future. Or, as suggested by Baumgartner and Jones (1993, 2002; Jones, Sulkin, and Larsen 2003; Jones and Baumgartner 2005), does real policy reform require a punctuation in which comprehensive coverage laws rapidly diffuse across the states? Fourth, we are interested in how the vertical diffusion process worked in universal health care: How did the failure of President Clinton's health care plan proposal spur states on to develop their own plans? And how did the experiences of state health care plans, especially that of Massachusetts, affect the development of the ACA in 2010?

We investigate these issues by first reviewing the history of efforts to promote universal health care in the states. The next section constructs a model of policy activity on universal coverage based upon the model we have used throughout the book. The third section uses a unique fifty-state data set that records all instances of universal coverage policy activity beginning in 1988. We then estimate the model with these data from 1988 through 2002. The findings are discussed in the conclusion in terms of the effects of organized interests on this particular reform and the ability of incremental steps to achieve large reform goals.

A History of States and Universal Health Care, 1974–2012

Although most people probably think of single-payer plans when the term "universal health insurance" is used, when health policy experts employ the term it applies more generally to any effort to provide health insurance to *all citizens*.[2] As defined in this broad manner, every state has at least studied proposals that fall under the rubric of universal coverage. Such proposals state a goal of universal coverage and provide a comprehensive plan or at least a legal framework of voluntary and mandatory steps to be enacted, funded, and implemented. Operationally, our data sources—the Intergovernmental Health Policy Project (IHPP), now defunct, and the National Conference of State Legislatures (NCSL)—judged five types of legislation as fitting the definition of universal coverage. Some proposals focused on controlling the costs of health insurance by regulating the market; others mandated employers to cover their employees' health insurance. Another type of universal coverage legislation used state funds to set up health insurance programs for needy families and adults without children who do not qualify for Medicaid. In some cases, people of modest means can buy into the program by paying a sliding-scale premium. The more far-reaching programs combined all three elements—cost controls, employer mandates, and public funding. The most comprehensive system is a single-payer plan, but until 2011 none had been adopted by a state. Still, the states have taken various steps during the last four decades toward universal health care—even if, in the end, success remains elusive.

In 1974 Hawaii passed the Prepaid Health Care Act, the first mandatory, employer-based insurance system. Though passing the bill took three years of negotiation, it was not especially controversial in the end, according to the Senate majority leader (Ching 1980, 71). Interestingly, the motivation for the bill was that Hawaiian leaders thought the federal government and other states were about to enact compulsory health insurance, and Hawaii wanted to join the crowd (Neubauer 1997, 171). Hawaii's leaders' forecasts were off by a decade and a half as far as the states were concerned (Massachusetts was the next adopter in 1988), and three and a half decades off for the nation. So what happened to the state health reform parade that Hawaii intended to join, but ended up leading?

The next wave of state activity occurred between 1988 and 1993, when six more states adopted universal coverage: Massachusetts (1988), Oregon (1989), Florida (1992), Minnesota (1992), Vermont (1992), and Washington (1993). In the Bay State, Democrats wanted theirs to be the first state after Hawaii to enact universal coverage in order to help Governor Michael Dukakis win his party's presidential nomination (cited by Paul-Shaheen 1998, 335). Based on a play-or-pay employer mandate, the new law was opposed by the next governor, Republican William Weld, and was never implemented. It was repealed in 1996.

In 1989 Oregon became (in)famous for passing a law that "rationed" Medicaid benefits while extending them to all citizens below the federal poverty line (FPL). The chief author of the legislation was Dr. John Kitzhaber, then president of the state Senate and later governor, serving three nonconsecutive terms. A lesser-known companion bill with a play-or-pay employer mandate was also enacted. But play or pay was never implemented due to the lack of an Employee Retirement Income Security Act (ERISA) waiver and loss of political support by the time of the law's self-imposed 1996 implementation deadline.[3] The following year, however, the Oregon legislature adopted the Family Health Insurance Assistance Program, a fully state-funded program for both adults and families earning up to 200 percent of the FPL. Thus, after dropping its employer mandate, Oregon found a way to continue its commitment to universal coverage for at least some portion of the public.

The next set of states took action in 1992–93, when it appeared that universal health care reform might soon be enacted at the national level. Notably, Vermont committed to universal coverage in 1992 by adopting a global health care budget and establishing a public authority to present single-payer and multipayer universal access plans to the next legislative session. However, by 1994, political support for the proposals in the legislature had evaporated, and neither plan was enacted. Interestingly, lack of gubernatorial leadership by Howard Dean was cited as a contributing factor in the plan's failure (Leichter 1997b, 211). The following year, Governor Dean was able to get the Vermont Health Access Plan (VHAP) through the legislature. Among its features was an expansion of Medicaid coverage to all uninsured adults not otherwise eligible up to 150 percent of the FPL. On the basis of VHAP and other programs, NCSL classified Vermont as having universal coverage in 1995, even though it did not adopt its first universal coverage plan (NCSL 2005).

Reform in Florida was short-lived. In 1992 the legislature and Governor Lawton Chiles enacted the Health Care Reform Act, with a promise of universal coverage by 1994. The first step was managed competition based on voluntary community health purchasing alliances. However, in 1994, Senate Republicans rejected the companion bill providing coverage expansion for the uninsured and thereby left Governor Chiles in a weakened position in his reelection bid. Thus, Florida's reform plan fell apart when it came to funding it.

Minnesota's reform had a more long-standing impact. It began in 1992 with the passage of the HealthRight law (the program's name was soon changed to Minnesota Care). Unlike the gubernatorial genesis of universal care proposals elsewhere, this bill was crafted by legislative entrepreneurs, the so-called Gang of Seven, a bipartisan group from both houses of the state legislature. On the day of the bill's final passage, Republican governor Arne Carlson, earlier an opponent of universal coverage, personally rounded up votes on the floor of the House.[4] The law relied on managed competition and regulatory controls (later dropped) to contain costs and extended health care access to uninsured adults and families via the state-funded Minnesota Care program. In 1994 the legislature adopted a goal of achieving universal coverage by 1997, but the next year changed its mind and rolled back the goal. Nonetheless, the Minnesota Care program survived, and into the next decade "Minnesota boasts one of the nation's most expansive publicly funded health insurance programs" (Holahan and Pohl 2003, 202).

The last state in this wave of reform was Washington, which provided universal coverage in 1993 through an employer mandate and a state-subsidized health insurance program, the Basic Health Plan (BHP). Initially, employers could also purchase insurance through BHP by paying the full premium. But when adverse selection problems developed, the program devolved to one with eligibility limits. Even though the reform had originated in the legislature, by 1995 that body had rescinded its goal of universal coverage and dropped the employer mandate. But the BHP continued, covering families and childless adults up to 200 percent of the FPL.

In addition to the actions of these six states, Hawaii took further steps toward universal coverage in 1989 when the legislature adopted the State Health Insurance Program (SHIP), which was designed to provide health care coverage for individuals and families with incomes up to 300 percent of the FPL.[5] Recipients below the FPL paid nothing, and those above paid on the basis of a sliding scale. In 1994 SHIP and the Medicaid patient populations were folded into the QUEST program, which is run under a managed care model. Childless adults continue to receive state-only funds up to 100 percent of the FPL today, thus continuing Hawaii's long-standing commitment to incrementing toward universal access.

Although these seven states were the pioneers receiving the most attention, ten other states passed more limited versions of universal coverage laws. In 1993 seven states—Arizona, Colorado, Iowa, Maryland, North Carolina, Texas, and Virginia—enacted various types of cost control initiatives, some on a limited or experimental basis, as a prelude to adopting universal coverage laws. Kentucky did the same in 1994, and Maine and Utah joined them in 1996. Then the universal coverage movement seemed to run out of steam for a while.

The next burst of activity, at least in terms of completed legislation, was not until 2003, when Maine adopted its Dirigo Plan and California enacted an employer mandate. The latter was repealed by California voters in a ballot referendum the next year. The Dirigo Choice Health Plan ("Dirigo," the state's motto, means "I lead" in Latin) is a voluntary program for individuals with incomes below 300 percent of the FPL, for solo proprietors, and for small businesses (under fifty employees). Participants pay on a sliding scale according to income. The program was a campaign issue for Democrat John Baldacci, who was elected governor in 2002 and who had promised universal coverage in five years. Its impetus was the sharp increase in insurance costs between 1996 and 2001, not the increase in the number of uninsured people (Miller and Rosman 2004). The program got off to a shaky start due to funding and administrative problems. But by 2010 the plan was being administered successfully by the Harvard Pilgrim Health Care Plan, financing had been stabilized (thanks in part to new federal dollars), and enrollment had increased to more than 30,000 members. However, in November 2010 Tea Party Republican Paul LePage was elected governor, and he promptly announced that he planned to scrap the Dirigo health program. Its funding was reduced in the 2011 legislative session and became intertwined with the reduction of funding in the Medicaid program. The future path of each seems to depend upon the implementation of health insurance exchanges/marketplaces in 2014 under the ACA.

In 2006 Vermont enacted the Catamount Health Plan to offer state-sponsored insurance coverage, plus several other acts, which together were intended to control the rising cost of health care by better management of chronic disease and expanding access to all. Premiums are scaled according to the income of the recipient. Republican governor Jim Douglas worked out the details of this plan with legislative leaders, after he had vetoed a similar universal care plan two years before. Funding comes from Medicaid, tobacco taxes, and a play-or-pay fee imposed on employers. By the spring of 2010, Catamount Health was having financial difficulties, even though slightly less than half of the 47,000 uninsured Vermonters had signed up for coverage in this or other government programs (Vermont Campaign for Health Care Security Education Fund 2009). In 2011 the Vermont legislature passed and Democratic governor Peter Shumlin signed legislation, which set the state on a path toward a single-payer health system, the first in the nation. This system will be called Green Mountain Care and could be implemented as early as 2014 if adequate funding is secured and if the Obama administration grants a waiver for it to operate within the health insurance exchange. Otherwise, Vermont will have to wait until 2017, which is the first time the ACA, as passed, permits state experimentation.

Also in 2006 Massachusetts adopted a universal health care package, called Chapter 58, which relied on an individual insurance mandate, plus a play-or-pay provision for firms with more than ten employees. The ambitious goal was to cover 95 percent of uninsured residents by 2009, which was met a year early in the fall of 2008 when 96 percent were insured. The 2006 legislation was a bipartisan effort between the Republican governor, Mitt Romney, and the Democratic Legislature. They established Commonwealth Care, which provides subsidized coverage for people with low incomes who are not Medicaid-eligible. Next the state set up a new private insurance purchasing exchange, called the Connector, where people with somewhat higher incomes and employers can purchase insurance on an income-scaled basis. Of particular importance, the Massachusetts program early on got favorable media attention; it was successful in enrolling clients early and was even popular with the business community, according to a 2007 survey of employers (Gabel, Whitmore, and Pickreign 2008). More than 430,000 people have gained coverage, driving down the percentage of uninsured to the national's lowest (Sack 2009b). Still, Governor Deval Patrick, a Democrat, has had to focus much of his attention on controlling the costs of care in this successful program. Other issues are that insurance premiums continue to be too high for many people and adding so many people to the health care system at once creates access problems for everyone. Yet, despite these problems and the issues brought on by the recession, this health care program remains popular in Massachusetts, with public support averaging 69 percent between 2006 and 2009 (Long and Stockley 2010). Most important—and this is the main difference from the experience in the 1980s and the 1990s—Massachusetts and Vermont have not abolished their programs due to fiscal problems but have tinkered with them and improved them. The Massachusetts program even served as a prototype for President Obama's plan, as we discuss at the end of the chapter. In contrast, the Dirigo plan in Maine was running a surplus in early 2012 (Farwell 2012), but the governor proposed to transfer the surplus to the Medicaid program as part of his plan to dissolve Dirigo.

Although only seventeen states adopted any type of universal coverage legislation during our study period of 1988–2002, the states' involvement was much broader than the record of adoption indicates. At the peak of activity between 1992 and 1994, thirty-eight study commissions or task forces were appointed by state legislatures. A report from such a commission almost always preceded any legislation on the subject. Moreover, the interest in universal access was so widespread that all fifty states authorized study commissions at one time or another. Formal consideration of universal access legislation also peaked at the same time. Fully fifty bills on the topic were introduced

Figure 5.1 Discrete Number of Final Universal Coverage Policy Acts by Year, 1988–2002

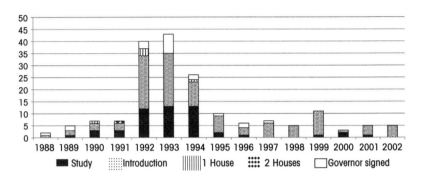

Source: Reprinted with permission from Gray et al. (2011).

in 1992 and 1993 (some states having more than one), tapering off to only ten in 1994 and nine in 1995. And forty-two of the fifty states had universal coverage bills introduced for consideration at some point. The states that were uninvolved tended to be southern (e.g., Louisiana) or small in population (e.g., Wyoming and the Dakotas).

At the same time states were considering and enacting universal health care legislation, the early adopters were already delaying implementation, were unable to enact the second phase of their legislative plans, or were repealing their laws. This amendatory phase of activity peaked between 1993 and 1996. Among the chief reasons for states' changes in plans were the fate of the Clinton health care reform package in Congress, the roadblock of the Employee Retirement Income Security Act (ERISA), and the states' own fiscal and political realities. The politics of state-level comprehensive reform were tied to expectations about similar reforms at the national level. We noted above that when Hawaii took action in 1974, and again when states began their reform efforts in the period 1988–92, it was with the expectation that national health insurance might soon be a reality; indeed, one book's title was *Five States That Could Not Wait* (Fox and Iglehart 1994). But as Clinton's reform package began to fail in the US Congress in late 1993 and finally died in 1994, the effect on comprehensive reform everywhere was devastating (Oliver and Paul-Shaheen 1997; Paul-Shaheen 1998, 355; Brown and Sparer 2001). Public support for universal health care eroded, and the drop in state legislative activity reflected that sentiment. The number of laws enacted from 1994 on declined to one or two per year, as did the number of universal coverage studies after 1994. The number of bill introductions after 1994 declined to four or five per year. Clinton's failure chastened state legislators as well as members of Congress.

ERISA's language appeared to preempt play-or-pay laws and other employer mandates. So, typically, states would make the implementation of such laws contingent upon receiving an "ERISA waiver," which Congress never granted. Consequently, universal coverage laws based on employer mandates either expired or were repealed in state after state. Because states could not force employers to provide employees with health care benefits, the burden of providing universal coverage fell upon the public sector, where it competed with other priorities in the regular budget process.

Moreover, by the early 1990s, most states were experiencing a recession, which made budgeting for significant new financial commitments unrealistic, and by 1994 there was a Republican upsurge in many states. Among the consequences for universal health care reform was that some of the early adopters dropped out when the price tag of universal access became apparent (e.g., Massachusetts and Florida). And the recession meant that new adopters in the mid-1990s tended to focus exclusively on controlling health care costs before making spending commitments (e.g., Kentucky in 1994, Utah in 1996). Comprehensive reform was out and incrementalism was back in. Not until 2003 would another state enact some form of universal health care.

Measurement of State Activity

In the following analysis we focus exclusively on those *state-funded* policies described above rather than joint state–federal programs such as Medicaid or the Children's Health Insurance Program (CHIP). Research has shown that redistributive programs funded solely from state coffers are the products of a different kind of politics than programs receiving funds from the national government (Barrilleaux and Bernick 2003; Barrilleaux and Brace 2007). Moreover, we are interested in programs whose explicit goal is universal coverage, not targeted coverage of a specific population. Programs aimed at covering the entire population—young and healthy uninsured people, workers who do not have employee coverage, and the uninsurable, along with the near-needy, while retaining the employer-based insurance system—have very different issues from programs that target a specific population. But certainly we acknowledge that states have also sought to expand health access through use of the Medicaid program, especially its Section 1115 waiver program, and by placing low-income children in the CHIP program.

Since no state in our data period of 1988–2002 has completed the policy cycle such that it can claim to provide full comprehensive care for all its citizens, our dependent variable cannot be the simple one or zero typical of state policy innovation studies. Rather, we measure the level of policy activity in a state moving toward the goal of universal health care, highlighting the various kinds of universal coverage policies noted above—cost controls, employer mandates, state-funded insurance programs for the near-needy, combined programs, and single-payer plans. An unusually wide array of sources—listed in appendix 5.1—was used to identify these policy activities and the ultimate fate of individual proposals.[6] Of particular importance, we relied heavily on two expert and reliable sources—IHPP and NCSL—to identify which bills fit the definition of universal coverage. Bills for three years come from IHPP and for ten years come from NCSL. Using their definition, the senior author identified universal health care bills from the Lexis/Nexis Bill Tracking database for four years. With the assistance of staff members at IHPP and NCSL, we were able to piece together systematic information on all universal coverage legislation considered in all fifty states back to 1988. Thus we are able to include in our data set all but Hawaii's first enactment.

We focus specifically on five levels of legislative activity, scored from one to five in terms of their proximity to the final goal of delivering universal access: (1) commissioning a study on universal coverage; (2) either introduction of a bill in the legislature to establish a program, set a goal of universal coverage, initiate the process of amending the Constitution, or call for a referendum on universal coverage or other evidence of significant legislative activity, such as a committee hearing; (3) passage of a bill by one chamber of the legislature; (4) passage of a bill by both houses; and (5) signing of the bill into law by the governor. We argue that higher scores on this continuum demonstrate greater legislative support for the policy proposal of universal coverage.[7]

We necessarily made a number of simplifying assumptions in coding these activities. First, each policy activity was coded only once, at the furthest point along the policy process that it managed to proceed within one year. Thus, a policy event coded four for passage in both houses supersedes its coding for passage in one house or reliance on a prior commissioned study within that year. So, if there was both a bill and a study within a calendar year, the bill was coded, but not the study, on the principle that the higher-order activity was the most noteworthy. Second, sometimes, although not very often, more than one bill was introduced within a single year. We initially coded both bills, but

Figure 5.2 Weighted Number of Final Universal Coverage Policy Acts by Year, 1988–2002

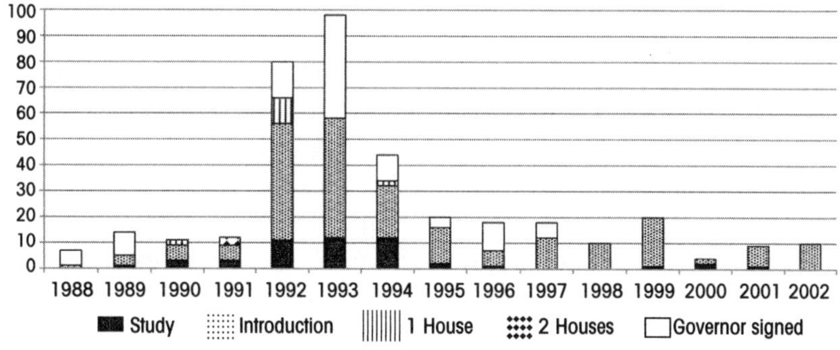

Source: Reprinted with permission from Gray et al. (2011).

count only the one that went furthest toward completion of the policy cycle, again based on a higher-order principle. Third, for the sake of simplicity, we assume that policy activity in each year is independent of activity in other years. Thus, in states with carryover provisions, a state that passes a bill in one chamber in one year and the other in the following year will receive a policy activity score of three for the first year and a score of four in the second. The main effect of this assumption is that it may bias our results toward finding evidence that policy activity in one year promotes greater activity in the next. We will see, however, that this potential source of bias has little impact on our findings.

The aggregate distribution of policy activities was already reported in figure 5.1. The values there were the number of discrete, highest-order events for all states in each year from 1988 to 2003. In figure 5.2 we take these values and weight the policy events from one to five in terms of how far along in the policy process they proceeded. Focusing on either discrete or weighted policy events demonstrates the same boom-and-bust cycle. From a near standstill in policy activity in 1991, a majority of states engaged in some level of activity in 1992, 1993, and 1994. Most of these were at the early stages of the policy process—commissioning a study and bill introductions or related activity. But a handful of states successfully passed legislation in one or both houses, and several adopted laws promoting universal coverage. New policy activity declined markedly after 1994, although a handful of policy events occurred each year.

We also employ a second version of the policy event measure in order to take account of variations in the *scope* of the proposals legislatures considered.

The scope of government involvement likely affects the probability of the proposal being enacted because a policy of wider scope will affect more interests and hence is less likely to be adopted. Empirically, the scope of proposals ranged from (1) cost control initiatives such as managed competition, voluntary purchasing alliances, or state-negotiated insurance rates in the context of a plan for universal health care; (2) mandates on employers to purchase health insurance for their employees or play-or-pay proposals that create incentives for employers to provide health insurance, both scored two; (3) *state-subsidized* insurance programs for adults and children above a certain percentage of the FPL and not covered by Medicaid, coded three; (4) mixed public–private proposals, including managed competition or employer mandates and *state-subsidized* health insurance for near-needy adults and children, scored four; and (5) a single-payer plan. Thus the level of government involvement expands as the scale increases from one to five. Each bill was assigned a scope score, but studies were not rated on this dimension because they were often wide-ranging in focus. These scores were multiplied by the level of policy activity variable to produce an alternative dependent variable weighted by the scope of the proposal under consideration.[8]

Of particular importance, to be included in our study, bills must be conceived as part of a plan for or step toward insurance coverage for all citizens. For this reason Medicaid expansions such as TennCare are not counted because they cover only certain categories of needy populations.[9] Figure 5.3 displays the policy event scale as multiplied by policy scope and shows the tremendous surge in number and magnitude of scope of policy proposals in 1993, reaching its zenith in 1994, and falling rapidly thereafter, though some activity continued until 2002.

Modeling State Policy Activity

Our theoretical expectations are drawn from the several sources explained in chapters 1 and 2. We will use the same basic model as employed in chapters 3 and 4, examining the influence of interest groups as well as variables measuring problem severity or need for the policy, political context, policy diffusion, and state capacity. Another source of our hypotheses is the extensive case study literature that highlights the early adopters of universal coverage and their role in promoting later actions by other states (e.g., Fox and Iglehart 1994; Leichter 1997a; McDonough 1992; Hackey and Rochefort 2001; special issue of *Journal of Health Politics Policy and Law* 2004). A close reading of chapters in these edited collections shows certain commonalities among the early

Figure 5.3 Weighted Policy Events * Policy Scope, 1988–2002

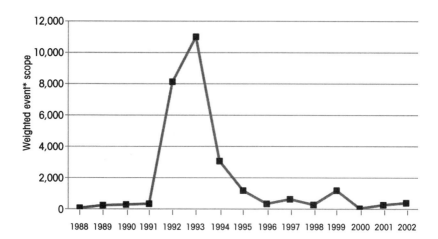

Source: Calculated by the authors.

adopting states. They tended to be liberal, wealthy, controlled by Democrats, and have several health maintenance organizations (HMOs) operating within the state; these are all variables that point toward an internal determinants version of policy innovation. Relatedly, a smaller number of studies attempt to synthesize findings of case studies or focus some other analytic lens on the path of universal access reform. Perhaps the best example is a lengthy article by Pamela Paul-Shaheen (1998). On the basis of the experiences of seven states, she concludes that policy entrepreneurs and the support of key stakeholders (interest groups) as well as the right window of opportunity are particularly crucial (see also Oliver and Paul-Shaheen 1997; Gold et al. 2001).

Our estimating models include five sets of independent variables, which are familiar by now from earlier chapters; the data sources for all these measures are reported in appendix 5.2.

Interest Organizations

The first set of independent variables is made up of organized groups that support universal coverage reform and organized interests that oppose it. At the national level the canonical story about health care policy reform in the early 1990s was about public interest waging an uphill struggle against the power of big interests. This story lies at the heart of the standard interpretation of the failure of President Clinton's national health care plan in 1994.

Many scholars (Jamieson 1994; West, Heith, and Goodwin 1996; West and Loomis 1999; Weissert and Weissert 2002; Quadagno 2005) and journalists (Johnson and Broder 1996) assigned primary blame for this fiasco to powerful interests representing the health care industry. Even scholars identifying other culprits—asserting that the president's strategy somehow "boomeranged" (Skocpol 1996) or that "It's the institutions, stupid!" (Steinmo and Watts 1995)—argued that one consequence of their preferred culprit's culpability was to yield enormous power to intransigent organized interests. Prior work on state health policy, however, has generated conflicting results on the role of organized interests. In chapter 4 we found strong results for advocates when examining how the composition of state interest communities influenced the adoption of managed care regulations during the 1990s, but puzzling results for enemies of regulation. Stronger results were found in chapter 3's examination of drug assistance laws, albeit again somewhat mixed; we found that the composition of state interest communities had little impact on the adoption of these laws, but a significant impact on their later revision.

We expect, however, that the structure of interest systems will matter a great deal for the success of universal coverage proposals. Such proposals entail either substantial state spending or the imposition of significant burdens on employers, alternatives that should take the debate over universal health care beyond the exclusive purview of health interest organizations to encompass a wide range of state interest organizations. Paul-Shaheen (1998, 329) argued that the cost crisis destabilized the existing health interest group system, long dominated by providers, and brought in business interests and consumer advocates. Fox (1994), in an analysis of the states that have promoted universal health care during the twentieth century, identified the important advocacy groups as labor unions, women's groups, and public interest groups.

A number of interests supported universal health care proposals in the 1980s and 1990s. First, health organizations, defined narrowly here to include those associated with the actual direct provision of health services, tend to favor expansion of health care coverage because they seem to think that health care is a good thing that should be available for everyone. This does not mean, of course, that all health care providers necessarily supported all efforts to promote universal coverage. Indeed, physicians and hospitals sometimes opposed universal coverage legislation. But when it became clear that reform would pass, organizations representing these interests often jumped on board. So, physicians and hospitals were often included in the coalition lobbying for the final passage of bills promoting some form of universal coverage short of single-payer systems (Paul-Shaheen 1998, 328). Their natural allies in this quest were liberal advocacy organizations attentive to the interests of the disadvantaged in society. Here, such interests are defined as civil rights, welfare, religious, environmental, and women's organizations.[10]

We believe that three and perhaps four types of organized interests opposed universal health care legislation. Small business and tax interests were clearly opposed to the proposals because of the actual or potential costs of universal coverage. Insurance interests were opposed because they stood to lose clients to state insurance pools or they would lose control over whom they could cover in their health insurance plans. Big business is more complicated. Big business—here defined as manufacturing, banking, transportation, and communication organizations—would certainly be unhappy with the cost of providing universal coverage via state spending of tax dollars or by employer mandates. But at the same time, a number of large businesses found the purchasing of health insurance for employees to be a significant burden as its cost rose to incorporate the uncompensated care provided to the uninsured especially in hospitals. Thus, a number of the largest businesses, either as individual firms or allied in employers' coalitions, began to support efforts to expand access to coverage as a means of obtaining a more level playing field in market competition especially in globally competitive markets. On balance, however, we expect that the cost argument may have prevailed over most of the period examined here, which would imply a negative coefficient in the model.

As before, we measure the structure of state interest communities by the number of lobby registrations by organizations representing these allies and opponents of universal coverage as a proportion of the total number of lobby registrations by interest organizations. Because such data are not available on an annual basis, our measures are the averages of 1990 and 1997 values of these variables. Thus, they vary only by state and not over time. Still, the 1990 and 1997 proportions are positively related to each other, suggesting that the relative strength of organized interests in terms of representation within state communities of organized interests is somewhat stable. But these correlations are not so high as to fully discount the importance of annual variations in influencing policy outcomes.[11] To anchor our proportional measures, the estimating models also include as a control the total number of organizations registered to lobby. Because values of this measure are related to the size of state economies, this variable will serve a second purpose of controlling for variations in consideration of universal coverage laws associated with state size.

Diffusion

A second set of independent variables is especially important given our interest in the sources of ideas about the universal coverage innovation. Consistent with the analysis of the extensive literature on interstate policy diffusion (Walker 1969; Gray 1973), does progress toward universal coverage in one state make it more likely that its neighbors will take policy actions promoting universal coverage? We measure this tendency by the lagged level of neighbor state policy activity. Among those who have written about the diffusion of comprehensive health reform in this incremental fashion are Leichter (2004) and Brown and Sparer (2001). Or is state policy diffusion in this area more governed by what is happening at the national level, given the case we made above for the connection of the states' consideration of universal care with the rise and decline of Clinton's universal health care plan? Our measure here is comparable to those used earlier: the lagged number of newspaper stories appearing across the country on the topic of "universal health care," "universal health insurance," or "universal health access."

Figure 5.4 shows that the number of stories about universal health care indeed spiked in 1994, coinciding with discussion of Clinton's plan in Congress. Stories then declined, only to spike again at a lower level in 2000, probably due to debate in the presidential election of that year. The next burst was in 2003, when our data series ends; this was the year in which state activity on universal care began again, with the adoption of the Dirigo Plan in Maine and an employer mandate in California, later repealed by the voters. This data series is modestly correlated at +.30 with the discrete number of policy events presented in figure 5.1, but the real question is how the national diffusion relationship holds up in a multivariate model.

The Political Context

Our third set of variables includes several measures of the political context in which proposals promoting universal coverage were considered. The first is state ideology, as captured by Erikson, Wright, and McIver's measure of public opinion liberalism.[12] Ideology seems to have played a somewhat varied role in state health policy during the last two decades. Barrilleaux, Brace, and Dangremond (1994) found state ideology (as measured by ADA scores) to be the strongest predictor of a set of health policy reforms adopted by 1994. In chapter 3 we found that opinion liberalism was strongly associated with the adoption of pharmaceutical assistance legislation, but it had little impact on the adoption of anti-HMO regulations in chapter 4. Paul-Shaheen (1998)

Figure 5.4 Number of Newspaper Stories on Universal Health Care, 1987–2003

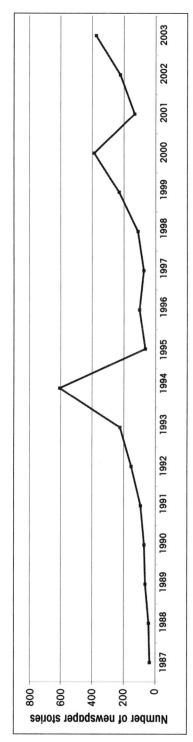

Source: Calculated by the authors from Lexis/Nexis.

identifies Democratic Party support as being key to initiating comprehensive coverage reform, but also stresses the importance of Republican collaboration for long-term success of the program. We measure partisan control with a dichotomous variable scored 1 if the governor was a Democrat, and the average of the two dichotomous variables for control of the two houses of state legislatures, again with nonzero values indicating partial or complete Democratic control. Last, interparty competition is a variable that is important to take into account in our explanation of an innovation. Pracht (2007) discovered that the more evenly competition was divided between the state's two political parties, the more likely it was that its Medicaid plan had embraced managed care. Interparty competition was measured by the folded Ranney Index, the standard measure in state politics research, with high values indicating higher levels of interparty competition.

Capacity

The fourth set of variables addresses the capacity of states to either adopt expensive new programs on their own or, instead, to impose costs on businesses. We expect that wealthier states will be more likely to do both. Grogan (1993) in particular has argued that only relatively wealthy states can afford to be innovative with respect to health care. State wealth is measured by per capita gross state product. We also examine the states' fiscal capacity more directly with the percentage annual change in total state revenue. States with growing budgets should be more inclined to adopt costly new programs. As noted above, blame is often assigned to the recession of the early 1990s in accounting for the ultimate failure of most states to accomplish universal coverage. State revenues should decline in periods of recession and fewer new programs should be adopted; existing programs may be disbanded or shrunk to the point of ineffectiveness.

Problem Severity

The fifth set of variables addresses the severity of the health care crises facing the states that would motivate policymakers to undertake universal coverage. Specifically, we employ four indicators—all of which are included as lagged values—addressing different health policy problems prominent in the universal coverage debate. The first two measures concern the cost of health care—the annual percentage increase in total health care costs and the per capita cost of drugs, both lagged. We think that efforts to promote universal health care will intensify when drug costs are high and when the overall cost of health care is increasing more rapidly. Paul-Shaheen (1998, 326) and

Oliver and Paul-Shaheen (1997, 756) identified escalating health care costs as the central "crisis" motivating comprehensive reform, but they emphasized that the perception of a crisis, not necessarily its reality, served as the catalyst. Such perceptions differed across the states. More important, however, efforts to promote universal coverage directly represent the lack of insurance coverage available to some citizens. The access issue had long been on the states' policy agendas, but usually of interest only to liberals. The cost crisis, particularly the cost-shifting of uncompensated care to business, brought conservatives to the table. Thus, we expect greater efforts to guarantee universal access in states with more uninsured citizens, as measured by the proportion of the population under age sixty-five who are uninsured.

Our last indicator of health policy problems is the proportion of the population enrolled in HMOs, a key measure of the structure and organization of the health care market being reformed. We have more mixed expectations about how HMO penetration may affect the prospects for universal coverage reform. Early in the period, both liberals and conservatives viewed HMOs quite positively as a prime solution to the perceived crisis in the costs of health care. It is clear that the few states that have traveled furthest toward universal coverage—Hawaii, Minnesota, Oregon, and Massachusetts—also had high rates of HMO participation. In these states HMOs were able to manage costs, which pleased businesses and led to higher rates of insurance coverage in the working population. Faced with smaller pools of uninsured individuals these state governments were able to extend coverage to the rest of the population by placing them in cost-effective HMO plans. From this perspective, higher levels of HMO penetration should lead to more universal health care activity.

But the severe backlash against diminishing choice and deteriorating services provided by at least some HMOs developed by the mid-1990s, and enrollments dropped by the end of the decade. Based on this scenario, the coefficient on HMO penetration should be negative. So it is unclear if high levels of HMO penetration should be considered part of the problem or part of the solution to the health care crisis. Our instinct is to opt for the latter interpretation—that HMOs on the whole facilitated the extension of universal health coverage—and therefore we predict a positive sign on this coefficient.[13]

Estimation

The models are estimated with data from 1988 through 2002 due to the limitations of our interest group data series; thus adoptions in Maine in 2003, in Vermont and Massachusetts in 2006, and in Vermont again in 2011 cannot be included in our data analysis though we discuss these laws further in

Table 5.1 Ordered Logit Analyses of Determinants of Weighted Universal Coverage Policy Events, Pooled 1988–2002 (n = 750)

Variables	Policy Event		
	Model 1.1	Model 1.2	Model 1.3
Interest organization variables			
Percent big business lobby of total lobby	.001	.000	−.014
	(0.03)	(0.00)	(−0.35)
Percent small business lobby of total lobby	−.081	−.085*	−.101*
	(−1.20)	(−1.25)	(−1.45)
Percent insurance lobby of total lobby	−.055	−.056	−.074*
	(−0.95)	(−0.97)	(−1.26)
Percent tax group lobby of total lobby	−.419*	−.410*	−.479**
	(−1.57)	(−1.54)	(−1.75)
Percent direct provider lobby of total lobby	.083**	.083**	.041
	(1.76)	(1.75)	(0.85)
Percent liberal advocacy lobby of total lobby	.069	.064	.037
	(1.18)	(1.10)	(0.62)
Total number of lobby registrations	.0007##	.0007##	.0007##
	(2.49)	(2.48)	(2.52)
Policy diffusion variables			
Lagged number of newspaper stories	—	.001**	.0003
		(1.70)	(0.41)
Lagged level of neighbor policy activity	—	—	3.43***
			(5.86)
Political variables			
Public opinion liberalism	−.634	−.450	−4.75
	(−0.62)	(−0.44)	(−0.45)
Folded Ranney index	.565	.569	.309
	(0.49)	(0.49)	(0.26)
Democratic governor	.375**	.378**	.329**
	(1.99)	(2.00)	(1.70)
Democratic legislature	1.01***	1.04***	1.08***
	(3.81)	(3.66)	(3.97)
Capacity variables			
Per capita GSP	.0002	.0002	.000
	(0.70)	(0.65)	(0.80)
Percent change in state revenue	.292**	.297**	.296**
	(2.18)	(2.25)	(2.25)

Table 5.1 *(continued)*

Need variables			
Lagged pct. increase in per capita drug costs	−.004	−.004	−.003
	(−3.00)	(−3.08)	(−2.27)
Lagged HMO penetration	2.55	.219	.346
	(0.24)	(0.21)	(0.32)
Lagged pct. population < 65 uninsured	−.046	−.048	−.061
	(−1.67)	(−1.72)	(−2.14)
Lagged annual pct. increase in total health care costs	−.029	−.011	.029
	(0.74)	(−0.27)	(0.69)
Ancillary parameters			
Cut 1	2.15	2.28	1.38
Cut 2	2.60	2.73	1.86
Cut 3	4.41	4.54	3.73
Cut 4	4.68	4.81	4.00
Cut 5	4.73	4.87	4.05
LR chi-square	71.16	73.97	108.16
Prob > chi-square	0.000	0.000	0.000

Note: Coefficients are standardized; z statistics in parentheses.
* $p < 0.10$, ** $p < 0.05$, *** $p < 0.01$, one-tailed test with robust standard errors clustered on states.
# $p < 0.10$, ## $p < 0.05$, ### $p < 0.01$, two-tailed test with robust standard errors clustered on states.

Source: Calculated by the authors.

the conclusions. Selecting an estimation method was more difficult than is usual for state policy studies. This difficulty in part results from the unfinished agenda on universal coverage. No truly comprehensive universal coverage policy was adopted by any state during this period, although Hawaii did so earlier. Rather, we are measuring policy events that take steps toward universal coverage. And because the scope of the proposed legislation varies and legislative sessions typically ended before the policy cycle was completed, finishing one step in the process does not mean that it will not have to be repeated for the same proposal or for another with a different scope. Thus, the states do not "drop" from the sample after completion of a given policy event as is typical of survival models or event history analyses. Nor do the data conform to the structure typical of count models. States may, for example, pass bills and implement one or more policies associated with universal health care, as is superficially typical of count models. But once a state passes and implements

Table 5.2 Ordered Logit Analyses of Determinants of Weighted Universal Coverage Policy Events*Policy Scope, Pooled 1988–2002 (n = 750)

Variables	Policy Event*Policy Scope		
	Model 2.1	Model 2.2	Model 2.3
Interest organization variables			
Percent big business lobby of total lobby	.073	.073	.065
	(1.49)	(1.48)	(1.29)
Percent small business lobby of total lobby	−.108*	−.109*	−.132*
	(−1.30)	(−1.32)	(−2.01)
Percent insurance lobby of total lobby	−.124**	−.124**	−.141**
	(−1.66)	(−1.66)	(−1.86)
Percent tax group lobby of total lobby	−.680**	−.678**	−.704**
	(−2.06)	(−2.05)	(−2.11)
Percent direct provider lobby of total lobby	.128**	.127***	.099**
	(2.27)	(2.26)	(1.71)
Percent liberal advocacy lobby of total lobby	.140**	.139**	.118**
	(1.96)	(1.93)	(1.61)
Total number of lobby registrations	.0007##	.0007##	.0007##
	(2.18)	(2.18)	(2.00)
Policy diffusion variables			
Lagged number of newspaper stories	—	.0004	−.000
		(0.59)	(−0.11)
Lagged level of neighbor policy activity	—	—	2.60***
			(3.82)
Political variables			
Public opinion liberalism	.266	.336	.246
	(0.21)	(0.26)	(0.19)
Folded Ranney index	2.40**	2.42**	2.14*
	(1.67)	(1.68)	(1.48)
Democratic governor	.427**	.424**	.414**
	(1.87)	(1.86)	(1.78)
Democratic legislature	1.08***	1.09***	1.12***
	(3.34)	(3.37)	(3.42)
Capacity Variables			
Per capita GSP	.000	−.000	−.000
	(−0.24)	(−0.25)	(−0.07)
Percent change in state revenue	.149	.149	.129
	(1.25)	(1.25)	(1.04)

Table 5.2 (*continued*)

Need variables			
Lagged percent change in per capita drug costs	−.002	−.002	−.001
	(−1.22)	(−1.24)	(−0.75)
Lagged HMO penetration	2.26**	2.24**	2.45**
	(1.75)	(1.74)	(1.86)
Lagged percent population < 65 uninsured	−.036	−.036	−.042
	(−1.07)	(−1.08)	(−1.24)
Lagged annual percent increase in total health care costs	−.035	−.028	.008
	(0.75)	(−0.57)	(0.15)
Ancillary Parameters			
Cut 1	7.08	7.14	6.59
Cut 2	7.22	7.28	6.73
Cut 3	7.37	7.43	6.88
Cut 4	7.43	7.49	6.94
Cut 5	7.78	7.84	7.30
Cut 6	7.80	7.86	7.31
Cut 7	12.12	12.18	11.63
LR chi-square	66.17	66.52	80.49
Prob > chi-square	0.000	0.000	0.000

Note: Coefficients are standardized; z statistics in parentheses.
* $p < 0.10$, ** $p < 0.05$, *** $p < 0.01$, one-tailed test with robust standard errors clustered on states.
# $p < 0.10$, ## $p < 0.05$, ###$p < 0.01$, two-tailed test with robust standard errors clustered on states.

Source: Calculated by the authors.

a law of a given scope, it need not do so again, something not easily assessed in count models. Thus, the most conservative estimation method is a simple pooled model using robust standard errors clustered on states. Finally, the models are estimated with logistic regression given the ordinal character of the policy event data that are our dependent measures, whether or not they are weighted by the scope of the policy.[14] One-tailed tests are used, except where we have already noted competing expectations.

Findings

The results reported in table 5.1 employ weighted policy events as the dependent variable. As discussed above, this variable measures final policy activity in each state-year and ranges from a commissioned study scored one to the governor's signing a bill into law scored five.

The dependent variable in the models in table 5.2, as also discussed above, uses these values multiplied by the scope of the proposal, giving us a fuller measure of the impact of the bill on the health industry. We therefore concentrate on the results in table 5.2. Although both dependent variables often generated similar results, we will note differences as they occur. Each table presents three models designed to test the sensitivity of the findings to inclusion of the external policy diffusion variables. Model 1 in both tables, the baseline model, omits all diffusion variables; Model 2 includes the national diffusion variable; and Model 3 includes the interstate diffusion variable as well as the national variable.

The relative sizes of the different organized interests supporting and opposing policy activity on universal health care generated our strongest set of findings. As seen in table 5.2, states with greater proportions of liberal advocacy interests and organizations representing direct providers of health care tended to promote universal coverage more; states with smaller proportions of small business groups, fewer advocates of low taxes, and fewer insurance interests were more likely to be further along the path to universal coverage, all as predicted by our theory. Another interest community variable—the total number of lobby registrations—was included more to anchor the other, proportion-based indicators of the relative sizes of different sectors of organized interests than to reflect a specific interest-based hypothesis. But given the strong relationship between number of lobby registrations and state size (Gray and Lowery 1996), the positive and significant estimates for this variable are best interpreted as indicating that larger states were more likely to be active on universal coverage than were smaller states.

But the weakest of these results was for the relative size of the big business sector, where none of the estimates were significant, and in table 5.2, all were positively signed contrary to expectations. As noted above, large businesses have quite mixed incentives with regard to promoting universal access, depending on whether they are ERISA-exempted or not, whether the proposed reform is market-based or regulatory, and so on. This is a level of nuance not applicable for the other subsets of organized interests. Overall, the results for the organized interest sector suggest that the organized advocates of universal coverage have considerable clout over the ability of universal coverage bills of increasing substance to get through the legislature and the opponents have contrasting sway over stopping such bills.[15]

In the introduction we stressed the seeming temporal relationship between the failure of President Clinton's health reform plan in 1994 and the collapse of health reforms in universal care by the states. However, the lack of significant results for the policy diffusion variables in table 5.2 demonstrates that overall the media's coverage of the universal health issue did not propel individual states to address the problem of universal access with their own policy proposals of increasing scope, once other variables are controlled for. However, model 1.2 of table 5.1 provides evidence of a positive and significant relationship between the number of media stories on universal care and promotion of universal care, as predicted. So there is an effect for the original variable before it is weighted by policy scope.

By far the stronger diffusion effect comes from the level of policy activity by neighboring states. In both tables if bordering states have considered proposals for universal health coverage involving a broader policy scope, then one's own state is more likely to do the same. This is a very strong relationship (significant at the .001 level), and it is an important demonstration of the continuing impact of state neighbors on policy activity. Apparently, incrementalism undergirds this area of policy diffusion in much the same way as it does for many other policy adoptions (Walker 1969).[16] Moreover, our finding reinforces that of Yackee (2009), who found interstate diffusion to be a strong predictor of medical malpractice reform, yet another politically salient health policy.

Strong results were also generated for most of the political context variables. Like our prior study of managed care regulation in chapter 4 (but unlike our study of senior drug assistance programs in chapter 3), efforts to promote universal health care during this period were far more a partisan issue than an ideological one. In table 5.2 none of the estimates for public opinion liberalism are significant (and in table 5.1 they are even wrongly signed). Democratic control of the governor's office matters a great deal, however, and legislative control by Democrats matters even more, with Democratic control positively associated with greater policy activity of a higher scope. Thus, our results on policy consideration during a fifteen-year time span underscore the observation of many that Democrats are usually in control when universal care policies are adopted (Paul-Shaheen 1998). The level of interparty competition also matters for predicting the scope of universal care proposals, as seen in table 5.2. These results mean that universal coverage policy considerations of broader scope get further in states marked by close competition between the two political parties for all offices.

Looking at state capacity as a predictor of policy consideration, we find that state wealth matters less than anticipated. The estimates for gross state product in table 5.2 were at zero, providing no additional information to explain states' universal coverage policy activity. Additionally, annual change in state revenues generated positive but insignificant estimates in table 5.2, implying that consideration of universal care proposals varying by scope is done without regard to changes in state revenue either. We do find, however, that the initial consideration of universal reform bills is predicted by the trend in the state's revenue stream, as shown in table 5.1 by the positive and significant coefficients. So, with a few exceptions, there is rather slim evidence to suggest that states are more active in promoting universal health care in good budget years than in lean. Surprisingly, most of the evidence suggests that states consider these proposals in both fat and lean budget years. But it may be that states still wait until the fat years to enact such reforms.

Finally, the models provide little evidence that variations in policy activity on universal coverage are associated with policy need. The lone exception was lagged HMO penetration in table 5.2 where, in all three models, HMO penetration was positive and significant at the .05 level. This means that states with higher levels of HMO penetration were more likely to have greater levels of policy activity promoting universal coverage with broader policy scope. The positive coefficients are consistent with the general thrust of the literature. Volden (2006), for example, found that HMO penetration captures the leader states whose success is emulated in the CHIP program. Any government efforts to extend access, as long as it is not delivered through a governmental single payer, would expand HMOs' patient pools.

None of the other problem severity estimates support our hypotheses. Consideration of universal coverage is not necessarily driven by the rising costs of drugs or the rising costs of health care in general. Further, legislative activity does not seem to respond to the size of the population without insurance. Variation in policy activity on universal health care is not associated with variation in objective measures of the severity of the health care crisis in the states.

Conclusion

In this final section we summarize our empirical results and compare them with national-level results on the forces impeding health reform. Then we consider whether universal coverage can be achieved incrementally or only through a policy punctuation. Third, we discuss the states' actions on universal coverage since 2002. First, our results indicate that variations in efforts to promote universal coverage were not primarily due to variations in the severity of the health care crisis in the states. This does not mean, of course, that there was not (or is not) a health care crisis or that its severity does not matter for public policy. Indeed, we prefer to think that the several crises in health care—lack of access to medical care, uneven quality of care, and high costs—are likely so severe and so widespread that their level is sufficient in every state to prompt policy attention.[17]

Our empirical results suggest that something more than a policy problem is required to secure policy action. Two sets of variables found to be especially important are Democratic control of government and the configuration of organized interests located in a state. When Democrats control the governor's office and the state legislature and allied interests make up a larger share of the interest community, legislative activity on policies promoting universal health care is more likely to occur. By the same token, when opposing organized interests are in smaller proportions, more legislative activity occurs. To some extent, then, state efforts to promote universal coverage seem to be governed by the same set of forces governing national efforts to promote universal coverage. Democrats, not Republicans, led President Clinton's charge on comprehensive health care reform, and organized interests were widely credited with stopping it or helping to stop it. Fifteen years later, Democratic president Obama had to make compromises in order to overcome organized interests to get his health reform bill through a US Congress controlled (barely) by the Democrats. However, it seems that in the states advocacy interests mattered more than in Washington: They helped the Democrats put the issue of universal coverage on the agenda in forty-two of the fifty state legislatures, and they helped Democrats to enact versions of universal coverage for a time in several states.

Adoption of innovations in the era under study in this chapter peaked between 1992 and 1994 and ended with a final enactment in 1997; though legislative consideration never ceased, enactments were on hold until a new burst of activity began in 2003. The lull in legislative success on universal health care coincides with the sudden drop in Democratic fortunes and the sharp increase in Republican office holding that occurred at the state level as a result of the 1994 elections. Republicans went from holding eight legislative branches in 1992 to controlling nineteen state legislatures in 1994 and continued to be in rough parity with the Democrats until the latter's rebound in the 2006 elections. Erosion of Democratic gubernatorial control came slightly later. The Democrats' drop occurred between 1994 and 1996, when they went from holding twenty-nine governors' seats to having only eighteen seats. Although they started inching back up in the early 2000s, the

Democrats did not achieve a large rebound in governorships until 2008. The twin declines in share of legislative seats and governorships held by Democrats in the mid-1990s almost certainly played a role in bringing the state universal care bandwagon to a halt.

Other conditions were found to be important as well. Close competition between the two political parties was another political variable that had some effect in facilitating consideration of universal care. Evidently where competition is close, health care reform is an issue that merits active consideration on the policy agenda. Two structural conditions stood out as significant: The total number of registered lobby organizations, which we consider a proxy for state size, and the degree of HMO penetration. Larger states were more likely to consider and act upon universal care legislation, as were states with a high proportion of their citizens covered by managed care. HMO penetration in these models appears to be a proxy measure for willingness to reform the health care market in general. Success in managed care apparently made policymakers more willing to consider and sometimes act favorably upon universal health care.

Last, the level of policy activity by neighboring states also positively affects promotion of universal coverage in a state. States whose neighbors were considering or enacting universal care were more likely to also move along the legislative path toward enactment of the same. Because universal coverage is expensive and any steps toward that goal are likely to be contentious, emulation of a familiar neighbor is very helpful in lowering the political costs of adoption. Our finding in this regard is important because it stands out in contrast to the general tone of the health policy literature, which rarely considers the influence of other states (Miller 2005), or if it does, finds geographic neighbors to have no discernible impact upon policy adoption (Volden 2006, but see Yackee 2009).

Having reviewed the model's results, we turn to consideration of the question: Can universal health care reform be achieved incrementally, or does it require a punctuation or burst of policy reform? The key question is whether small or early efforts within a given state toward universal health care make it more likely to take more significant policy steps later on. Does incremental change "go" anywhere? Because all the states coded for policy activity in our data set considered universal coverage as a policy goal, presumably they envisioned taking further steps at some point. The broad outlines of the scholarly approach known as incrementalism are familiar: Policymakers prefer the status quo until a problem comes up that requires a change. Then they search, using a variety of shortcuts, until they find an acceptable solution to the problem;

subsequently, that solution is adopted, making for a policy that changes only gradually over time. Incremental policymaking is also dictated by a set of institutional constraints—parties, interest groups, governmental institutions, complexity of the problem, inadequacy of solutions—that tends to dominate the political process. A few scholars have written about the incremental nature of comprehensive health reform at both the national and state levels (Fuchs and Emanuel 2005; Leichter 2004; Brown and Sparer 2001). According to Fuchs and Emanuel (2005), the health care reforms so far have been incremental: Employer mandates, subsidies for the uninsured to purchase insurance, and managed competition plans are examples. The enactment of these plans, along with CHIP and expanded drug coverage for Medicare beneficiaries at the federal level, has not eliminated the large number of uninsured people. The authors believe comprehensive reform can only be achieved by the combination of personal mandates and subsidies, a single-payer system, or a universal health care voucher (Fuchs and Emanuel 2005). Others, such as Oliver and Paul-Shaheen (1997, 741), argue that sometimes incremental reforms in health care can help create opportunities for nonincremental change by building up the knowledge base, broadening the political resource base of reformers, and enhancing confidence in the feasibility of policy change, that is, by serving as a positive feedback loop.

The number of critiques of the incrementalist approach is vast, but the number of opposing theories is small. The opposing theory of most significance for the last two decades has been Baumgartner and Jones's (1993) punctuated equilibrium theory. Jones and Baumgartner (2005) have extended their 1993 theoretical framework to argue for a disproportionate information-processing model: Constant political pressure will produce little change until the pressure reaches a critical threshold, and at that point the degree of movement can exceed even the degree of pressure. Only then do you get policy punctuations. When Baumgartner and colleagues applied the punctuated equilibrium model to the passage of a broad range of new legislation, they discovered that the status quo tended to prevail in Washington. However, policy change did occur in 30 to 40 percent of their cases, and when it did, it was more likely to be a significant rather than a modest change (Baumgartner et al. 2009, 311). They interpreted these findings as support for the punctuated equilibrium theory of policy change rather than the incremental theory.

What health policy change is large enough to constitute a policy punctuation? If we base our answer on Fuchs and Emanuel (2005), adoption of a single-payer plan by a state would be one example. Thus, Vermont's action in 2011 could set off a positive dynamic feedback loop in which other states respond by trying to enact single-payer and other universal coverage programs on their own. Indeed, the Democratic governor of Oregon now wants to move beyond traditional Medicaid by setting up coordinated care organizations and folding state employees into them too; the Democratic governor of Montana seeks to use the same path to get to a universal coverage program (Kliff 2011). Fuchs and Emanuel's (2005) second example—the combination of state subsidies and mandates—is in essence the Massachusetts plan adopted in 2006. Or at the national level it is the Affordable Care Act of 2010. But Jones and Baumgartner (2005) also envision a policy punctuation to be during a dynamic period in which different political units surge toward adopting a new policy, perhaps influenced by changing media frames.

If reform requires a true punctuation in which policies promoting universal coverage policies of wider scope rapidly diffuse across the states, what might set that bandwagon in motion in the first decade of the 2000s after our study period ended? Given our results, perhaps a confluence of two or three events is necessary to overcome entrenched interests opposed to policy reform.[18] The first enabling event is a period of relative economic stability or growth in which states feel emboldened to adopt new spending programs. Second, the fundamental barrier of ERISA needs to be lifted in order for states to pursue universal care via means such as mandating employees' health care coverage. If only the first condition occurs, new programs will emphasize state subsidies. If only the second occurs, reforms will likely emphasis the regulatory route. If both occur, mixed systems are likely to emerge, like those adopted—but never fully implemented—in Minnesota and Florida in 1992 and Washington in 1993. The third facilitating event that, given our results, is necessary to set off a policy bandwagon is the election of Democrats.

Did these stars align? For several years it appeared that maybe, just maybe, Maine might have set off a new policy bandwagon in 2003 with the adoption of its Dirigo Plan. Vermont enacted its Catamount Plan in 2006, focused on costs of care, and in the same year Massachusetts adopted a universal health care package that relies on the individual mandate. Massachusetts' action as a large state, in particular, made other states take stock of their access and cost problems once again. The next year the governors of California (R), Illinois (D), and Pennsylvania (D) proposed sweeping plans to restructure health care in their states, though none finished the year with bills signed, due to an imbalance in their interest organization systems fueling intense opposition from insurance and other business lobbies that had more clout than in the smaller New England states (Sack 2007). Altogether seventeen state legislatures considered universal health access bills in 2007, according to NCSL (2007).

Figure 5.5 Weighted Number of Final Universal Coverage Policy Acts by Year, 2003–9

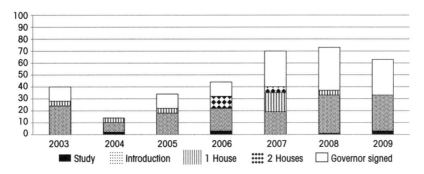

Source: Calculated by the authors.

Figure 5.6 Weighted Policy Events * Scope, 2003–9

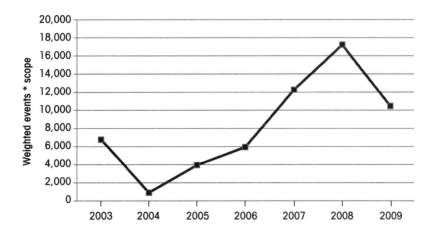

Source: Calculated by the authors.

Figures 5.5 and 5.6 display more systematically the types of activities states have engaged in since 2003. Interestingly, the number of states considering universal coverage bills seemed to grow over time, with 2007 through 2009 witnessing the most interest in universal care legislation. Certainly by the time of Barack Obama's election as president in late 2008, state policymakers knew he would attempt to enact a national comprehensive health care reform law, yet the states continued to press on with their own state solutions to the health care crisis throughout 2009. And the states did not just consider bills: Five states enacted universal coverage legislation in 2007, six in 2008, and five in 2009, for a total of twenty-two universal care enactments of some type from 2003 through 2009. However, it appears that the scope of the bills suddenly narrowed as legislatures got closer to the debate over the principles of President Obama's health care reform plan. The universal coverage bills multiplied by their scope had been increasing each year from 2004 through 2008, but then that number fell in 2009, indicating that the policy proposals being considered by state legislatures were narrower in their impact upon the health care industry and upon society.

What brought about this new boomlet? These events are outside the range of our study's reach, but we can note that Democrats regained state legislatures in 2006, going from seventeen in 2004 to twenty-four in 2006. Similarly, the number of Democrats occupying the governor's chair went from twenty-two in 2006 to twenty-eight in 2008, so the partisan political conditions were in place for universal health care to be on the agenda again. ERISA still had not been removed by the Congress, but states designed innovative ways around it: Massachusetts relied on an individual mandate, rather than on the employer mandate that had tripped it up in the late 1980s; Vermont made its program voluntary; and Maine financed its program initially out of savings generated from its cost controls.[19] Fiscal conditions were at least plausible in 2006 and 2007 for consideration of new large ticket items.

However, the surge in state health reform prospects of the early 2000s ran into the same trouble as did the programs we studied in the 1990s. The economy turned negative in the second half of 2008, which quieted states' enthusiasm for putting uninsured clients onto the state rolls, especially when a Democratic presidential candidate was campaigning to make health care universal if elected. The grim economic conditions of late 2008 and 2009 posed twin challenges for Massachusetts, Vermont, and Maine: The states had less money to spend on health care, but they had more clients in need of health insurance. Thus far, Massachusetts and Vermont have weathered this storm, arguably due to the support of the federal government, which provided fiscal relief under the American Recovery and Reinvestment Act and Section 1115 waivers that allowed states to continue to support health reform during a recession (Long and Stockley 2010). But these states' health plans, particularly that of Massachusetts, served more than just the residents of their own states. These health plans served as important touchstones for the Obama administration in crafting its ideas on health policy.

The Massachusetts plan's reliance on the individual mandate served as an important model for the Obama administration as it sought to draft its health care reform principles in 2009. Kingdon (2011, 237–38) stated that since the Massachusetts plan had been tested successfully in the real world, unlike proposals in Clinton's health reform package, it became a major model for the Obama plan. The requirement that every resident of the Commonwealth get insurance as well as the provision of state subsidies for lower-income people had proven quite popular; together they had resulted in coverage of most of the state's population. Both the individual mandate and subsidies are in the ACA. Likewise, the ACA has a requirement that employers of a certain size offer insurance to employees; the Massachusetts employer mandate was somewhat weaker due to ERISA.[20] In addition, the Massachusetts' Connector was an idea picked up by the Obama administration and became the model for its health insurance exchanges (Jacobs and Skocpol 2010, 90). Thus, the Massachusetts plan, which ironically had Republican roots with Governor Mitt Romney, was a model that would be emulated by Democrats in Washington via a vertical diffusion process. Both Paul Starr (2011, 206) and John McDonough (2011, 128) maintain that the Obama administration borrowed the idea of the individual and employer mandates and the insurance exchange from the Massachusetts plan. McDonough's account is particularly telling because he had worked on the Massachusetts plan, and he later served as staff to the Senate Committee on Health, Education, Labor, and Pensions (Senator Ted Kennedy's Committee) from 2008 to 2010. An analysis of White House meeting records showed that McDonough attended four White House meetings on the issue; also Jon Gruber, an economist at the Massachusetts Institute of Technology who advised the Romney administration on health care, attended five White House meetings in 2009 and he had a large contract to draft a new federal law based on the state law (Isikoff 2011).

Moreover, other states' experiences diffused upward as well. Since 1993 Maine had required sellers of individual health insurance policies to accept all applicants, a forerunner of the preexisting conditions clause of the ACA (Mathews and Johnson 2010). But negative experiences diffused upward as well as positive ones: Maine's Dirigo Plan was voluntary so insurers argued that an influx of sick customers drove their costs up beyond what could be recovered in premiums allowed by the state. The federal law's mandatory requirement that all obtain insurance was designed to fix that kind of problem.

The financial strains of Maine's and of Massachusetts' health plans made the Obama Administration acutely conscious of the need to present a health care reform bill that "could pay for itself" (Serafini 2009b). In fact, one of the primary motivations for tackling health reform was because the government's long-term debt problem was mostly due to the projected rise in health care costs (Kingdon 2011, 234). As 2009 turned into 2010, and the magnitude of the recession became clearer, the necessity for a cost-containment strategy became more critical. The federal cost-containment board in the ACA has significantly more authority than does the similar board in Massachusetts. In addition, important political lessons diffused upward from Boston to 1600 Pennsylvania Avenue: Front-load some of the benefits and delay the pain as long as possible was one of those lessons (Serafini 2009b). Thus, six months after the ACA was signed into law, a set of popular benefits kicked in, including coverage of adult children up to age twenty-six on parents' plans, no lifetime dollar limits on coverage, no preexisting conditions clause for children (and later for everyone), and coverage of preventive services, whereas the individual mandate does not take effect until 2014. The political strategy was to establish the plan first with the general public, gain their acceptance, and then add on the necessary mandates and taxes. Thus the experience of just a few states served as a guiding template for the Obama administration and an important demonstration of vertical federalism.

But the politics of vertical federalism was also working from the bottom up in a negative direction since 2010 as the American Legislative Exchange Council (ALEC) promoted its "Health Care Freedom Initiative" in state legislatures. ALEC is a conservative policymaking group which brings together state legislative members with corporate members and representatives from think tanks and foundations. Following the 2010 elections membership soared to 2000 legislators (Greenblatt 2011, 35). ALEC provided legislators with 18 model bills on health care, with the principal one, the "Freedom of Choice in Health Care Act," designed to push back against the ACA. This bill has been introduced in forty-four state legislatures, has been enacted as a statute in twelve states, and passed as a constitutional amendment in three states—Arizona, Oklahoma, and Ohio (American Legislative Exchange Council 2012). The legislation prohibits any person, employer, or health care provider from being compelled to purchase or provide health insurance and protects the right to pay directly for medical care. Passage as a statute is designed as a weapon against implementation of the ACA, while enactment of a constitutional amendment is crafted to prevent further state actions—such as a state individual mandate or a single-payer plan like Vermont's—if the ACA fails (American Legislative Exchange Council 2011, 12). Thus after passage of the ACA in March 2010 we began to see a shift in the political landscape: as more state legislatures, mostly under Republican control, expressed their displeasure with the federal law, they also turned away from the possibility of handling the access problem themselves, which states in general had been increasingly willing to do through 2009 (see figure 5.5). Because the Democrats retained control of the presidency and the US Senate, the ACA remains intact, and state health care reform will now proceed within its framework.

Notes

1. A number of scholars (e.g., West, Heith, and Goodwin 1996; Weissert and Weissert 2002; Jamieson 1994; West and Loomis 1999; Quadagno 2005) and journalists (Johnson and Broder 1996) assigned primary blame for President Clinton's health care fiasco to powerful interest groups representing the health care industry.

2. A single-payer plan is a government-run health plan with no private-sector involvement.

3. The ERISA roadblock dates back to 1974, when Congress enacted the Employee Retirement Income Security Act, which preempts state laws that "relate to" employee benefit programs (including health plans) unless such laws are part of the traditional state function of regulating insurance. This language would seem to preempt play-or-pay laws and other employer mandates. So, states typically made the implementation of such laws contingent upon receiving an "ERISA waiver." However, there was no process in federal law by which states could apply for such a waiver, and Congress never granted any such exemptions, Hawaii's law having been adopted before Congress acted on ERISA. So employer mandates either expired or were repealed in state after state.

4. This is an observation by one of the authors.

5. According to Oliver and Paul-Shaheen's (1997) analysis of the details of each state's health reform package, the components were largely developed in each state rather than borrowed as a complete package from another state.

6. We also coded a tiny handful of initiatives associated with universal coverage. But these could not easily be fit within our policy process model, which is focused on the legislative process. Still, there were very few initiatives, and none were successful.

7. Burstein, Bauldry, and Froese (2005) made a similar argument, using length of time on the congressional agenda and number of sponsors to measure support for policy proposals.

8. The two dependent variables are correlated at 0.69 so they are not measuring the same thing.

9. Likewise, Oliver and Paul-Shaheen (1997, 737n5) exclude TennCare from their set of cases because its plan lacks the scope of policy instruments of other states' universal coverage programs.

10. Labor unions constitute another set of obvious allies. However, the data

were not coded in a manner allowing us to separate out unions from the industries in which they work. Also, though sometimes very powerful, unions as organizations are remarkably small in number. Given our numerically based representation of the relative strength of organized interests, the inclusion of unions within their industries hardly alters those values. Still, unions constitute an unmeasured ally in our analysis.

11. For example, the correlation of the 1990 and 1997 proportions of insurance and liberal advocacy organizations are 0.67 and 0.51, respectively.

12. Values on this measure were missing for a handful of state-years, primarily for Alaska and Hawaii. Missing values were interpolated or, in cases where they occurred at the beginning or end of the time series, were assumed to have been unchanged from the last or next observed level of opinion liberalism at the beginning or end of the series, respectively.

13. The correlations among the health problem variables ranged from a low of 0.04 to a high of 0.42.

14. The product of policy event and policy scope that is used as the dependent variable in table 5.2 comes close to being interval. Indeed, estimation of these models with ordinary least squares regression generated essentially identical results. But given the uncertain metric between the policy event measures, the more conservative estimation strategy seemed to be continued reliance on logistic regression.

15. The results in table 5.1 are mainly in the correct direction, though of lesser or no significance.

16. One of the few studies to analyze legislative consideration separately from legislative adoption found interstate diffusion to be a significant positive predictor for consideration but not for adoption (Mintrom 1997). Another study compared the determinants of bill introductions with bill adoptions (Whitaker et al. 2012). They found that many of the traditional political and economic variables were significant for introductions but in the adoption model almost nothing worked.

17. The impact of universal coverage laws on the rate of the uninsured is a bit unclear. A study by Holahan and Pohl (2003, 208) compares leaders and laggards in universal coverage in the 1990s; their top tier of leaders includes the five states that implemented some form of universal coverage in the early 1990s—Vermont, Minnesota, Oregon, Washington, and Hawaii. This group of states used either state-only coverage or Medicaid to cover a larger proportion of the insurance gap for the total population, the low-income population, and the low-income adult population than did the three other groups of states. The only exception to this pattern of success was that the second tier of states came out slightly ahead on covering the insurance gap for low-income children (Holahan and Pohl 2003, 208), perhaps due to the effect of variations in usage of the SCHIP program.

On the other hand, Bernick and Meyers (2008) embedded forty-one states in a model comparing tax incentives versus twelve direct-coverage programs between

1995 and 2002, controlling for unemployment. The authors find that tax incentives provide no discernible relief for the uninsured in the states, while universal coverage programs that were state-sponsored yielded negligible results, when rising unemployment was factored into the model. However, federal efforts such as Medicaid and CHIP were successful in reducing the number of uninsured. One caveat to their study lies in the selection of the twelve state-only coverage states: only four of the states appear in our data set for the same period. Thus, we surmise that Bernick and Meyers (2008) may have included a number of state programs that were too minor to have much of an effect on the rate of the uninsured.

18. Fuchs and Emanuel (2005, 1412) seem much more pessimistic in that they envision the forces necessary for comprehensive reform in health care to be a major war, depression, or large-scale civil unrest, or perhaps a national health crisis such as a flu pandemic. Their conditions are more akin to what Baumgartner and Jones (2009, 285) have termed disruptive dynamics.

19. This offset savings element was challenged in court and eventually upheld by the Maine Supreme Court in 2007.

20. For a side-by-side comparison of the Massachusetts law, Chapter 58, and the ACA, see Patel and McDonough (2010, 1107).

CHAPTER 6

Conclusion

Lessons Learned and Opportunities for Influence in the ACA Policy Environment

In this final chapter we summarize our key findings about the role of interest groups in state health reform, comparing the three different reforms we have highlighted in this book. As noted in the introduction, this book is primarily one about the influence of organized interests with secondary emphases, albeit vital to a research design capable of addressing the first issue, on health policy and state policymaking. Thus, our conclusions bear on all three of these topics. In looking at the specific results, we first discuss the findings in terms of the innovation theory framework used throughout the book. Second, we consider why organized interests play a greater role in some policies than in others. Here we discuss how the Energy Stability Area (ESA) model contributed to our understanding of interest group activities. And third, we describe the states' critical role in implementing the Patient Protection and Affordable Care Act (ACA), both how well they are prepared to do the job, based on their previous experience as health care reformers, and how hostile some states are to cooperating with the federal government at all.

However, before considering these specific findings on our three topics of interest, it is important to note that perhaps our central finding on all of them concerns the heterogeneity of the results. That is, interest organizations were sometimes found to be influential and other times not. And the very definition of allies and enemies among organized interests changes from one health policy topic to another, and some of these policies were successfully adopted across the states and others not. Indeed, the determinants of successful policy adoption varied from one policy to another. In short, our findings offer a far more complex view of the influence of organized interests, their role in health policy debates, and the determinants of policy adoption than is common. Quite often, the sides taken on health policy issues or who is wearing the white and black hats are simply assumed on an a priori basis. From studies of a single issue, overly broad claims are too often made about the nature of the public policy process. In short, our findings do not offer a single simple conclusion about either the role of organized interests in health policy debates or their influence more generally.

Far from being a weakness, however, we view the heterogeneity of our findings as offering a useful corrective to several literatures by suggesting that the influence of organized interests, their role in the policy process, and the nature of state public policymaking are all highly contingent on the specific issue at hand. This has implications for both the literature on organized interests and claims about health policymaking. With regard to the former, in the broadest sense, this notion of contingency is most consistent with the neopluralist perspective introduced in chapter 1. In this view, organized interests can be highly influential at times and completely ineffective in others. Our findings highlight examples of both patterns of influence and help to assess when they are likely to be evident. And with regard to discussions of health policy, our results should go a long way in debunking the too-common story of the failure of health policy reform as "blame the interest groups." They proved to be neither monolithic in their policy preferences nor uniformly strong or influential across specific health policy reform proposals. In sum, the world is more complex than suggested by many who study the influence of organized interests and many who offer overly simple diagnoses about the process of making health care policy. Most especially, the specific nature of a given issue and its political context matter a great deal.

State Health Policy Reforms as Innovations

It has proven useful to frame our analysis of state health policy reforms as innovations and to pay attention to the way in which they diffused across the states. One—the attempt to curb managed care via regulation—was a movement that spread quickly across the fifty states; policymakers had only to leap on the bandwagon. Two others that involved more expenditures spread more slowly across the states and never involved all the states. But in the case of the two expenditure programs, we were able to conduct our analysis over time so that we could see the impact of external influences as well as internal determinants.

Internal determinants as a whole played a stronger role in explaining the patterns of state health reform than did external determinants. Partly, this finding may have been due to measurement issues; we could not measure the external influences on anti–managed care regulations because our design was cross-sectional. And our newspaper coverage variable did not capture all the national-level influences encouraging states to adopt the reforms. But overall, internal determinants were the better group of predictors. This is not to say that every set of internal variables contributed to the explanation. The measures of problem environment, or need for the policy, did not work as expected. Only for adoption and revision of state pharmacy assistance programs did need or severity of the problem matter very much, and in some of the anti–managed care models it mattered; it was not at all a factor in universal care consideration.

Measures of state capacity mattered for all three health policy reforms, though the exact measure of capacity differed. For consideration of universal coverage legislation (though not for scope of the coverage), it was change in state revenue that was significant and positive. For anti–managed care legislation, it was administrative capacity that mattered for both the number of regulations and their scope. For pharmacy assistance program adoptions, both wealth and change in state revenues mattered; capacity made little difference for revision and generosity for pharmacy programs, once they were established. Thus, it appears that the "slack resources" hypothesis about innovation was operative in these health care reforms, rather than the "necessity is the mother of invention" hypothesis.

Politics, broadly defined, played the most important role in the three health policy reforms. The varying impact of organized interests' politics is reviewed in the next section of this chapter; suffice it to say that interest organizations had a significant impact upon each of the three reforms, but the measures of interest organization differ across the reforms. Party politics had the greatest impact on consideration of universal coverage; both the number and scope of bills considered were significantly enhanced when Democrats controlled the state legislature and governorship. The politics of managed care regulation depended only upon Democratic control of the legislature, not the governorship, indicating that the legislative branch may be more interested in regulation than the executive branch. And for pharmacy assistance programs, party politics was critical only for the revision stage where the governor mattered more than the legislature. Close interparty competition also played a considerable role in expanding the scope of universal care proposals (though not their number), in increasing the number and stringency of regulations placed on managed care, and in the adoption (only) of pharmacy assistance programs. Thus, one can imagine that these were public programs promised when competition heated up between the political parties at election time.

The politics of health care reform in the 1980s and 1990s, however, seems to have been far more partisan than ideological in nature. Our ideology measure, public opinion liberalism, had no explanatory value for universal coverage or for anti–managed care regulation. It mattered only for adoption of pharmacy assistance programs, weakly for their generosity, and not at all for their revision. It is unclear why public opinion liberalism would perform so poorly; the measure is thought be to be relatively static across time, which would explain its poor showing in the time series models; however, it worked equally badly in managed care's cross-sectional model.

In the case of two reforms—pharmacy assistance programs and universal coverage—we were able to include measures of external determinants in our model. Both horizontal and vertical diffusion were evident. For consideration of universal coverage, horizontal diffusion was the important influence; states were likely to consider proposals more fully, and to contemplate ones of broader scope, if their neighbors had done so. The actions of a state's neighbors seem to pique the interest of policymakers in a state, but not enough to result in any adoptions of universal coverage. The impact of national news coverage on universal coverage consideration was also evident in the simple model, but not in the full model when external diffusion was included. In the case of pharmacy assistance adoptions, national news coverage was a significant influence in the full model; and to a milder extent this was true for the expansion of these programs. Horizontal diffusion did not play a significant role, however, in encouraging adoptions or revisions. As such programs received national media attention, the more likely they were to be adopted.

Due to the cross-sectional nature of the model used for anti–managed care regulations, we could not include measures of external influences in the model. Because the adoption of these regulations proceeded so quickly, it is likely that they might be subject to some of the same influences as the bandwagon policies studied by Nicholson-Crotty (2009), and the process can be categorized as a policy outbreak (Boushey 2010). Nicholson-Crotty (2009) found that policies that diffused rapidly were more likely to be highly salient, to be of low technical complexity, and to have been supported by other governors, among other things. He reasoned that in these circumstances little policy learning was going on. His seems an apt description of the swift reaction to the problems with managed care, the ease with which fairly simple solutions made it onto the policy agendas of most state legislatures, and their rapid passage. Few policymakers felt the need to wait for a full-scale evaluation of a policy's success in another state before regulating health maintenance organizations (HMOs) in their own states.

The diffusion paths of these programs have changed since our study period ended. The diffusion of pharmacy assistance programs was fundamentally transformed by the federal government's addition of Part D prescription drug coverage to Medicare in 2003. A few states dropped their programs; most states converted them to "wraparound coverage," but seven states did adopt their own new state pharmacy assistance programs. So states' commitment to their seniors continued after the federal government stepped in. The regulation of managed care is a different story: The first states enacted regulations in 1994, and less than a decade later, patient and physician rights were well established in the states. Diffusion was quick and then ceased; it involved all the states, but not the federal government. Our third policy—universal coverage—had a different diffusion path than either of these two: Adoptions began in Hawaii in 1974 and were fairly rare events, so rare that we studied consideration of universal coverage, not just adoption. But after the end of our study period, adoption of some type of universal coverage (as defined by the National Conference of State Legislatures) actually picked up the pace, with a total of twenty-two enactments between 2003 and 2009, including the three major examples in Maine, Vermont, and Massachusetts. The spread of the reform was then interrupted by the recession beginning in 2009 and adoption of the federal ACA in 2010. Aside from Vermont's adoption of a single-payer program, few states were likely to begin their own health plans after March 2010, given that they had their hands full implementing the new federal legislation, which gives them flexibility to establish a range of state health plans within their own insurance exchanges, now called marketplaces.

What about policy punctuations? The backlash against HMOs and its expression in the rapid diffusion of regulations across all fifty states is a classic case of a policy outbreak or punctuation. The new laws brought sweeping policy change characterized by a positive feedback cycle as all states adopted more than one of the anti–managed care regulations in a short period. It was as if a contagious disease had struck managed care plans and in less than a decade left behind much looser forms of health care networks. Universal coverage, in contrast, proceeded in fits and starts; its time path was characterized by two small spikes of adoptions, but most of the time we studied its consideration rather than enactment. The possibility of a policy breakthrough was halted by an economic recession, by changes in party control of state government, and more recently by the federal government's entrance into the policy space. Pharmacy assistance programs proceeded in a more incremental fashion, as is characteristic of the diffusion process of many less controversial, less salient policies (Boushey 2010); there was no sudden bandwagon.

The Role of Organized Interests in State Health Policy

The prevailing story that interest groups are responsible for stymieing health reforms in Washington is too simple a story to explain the effects of organized interests in the states across our three health policies. As discussed in chapter 1, the same organized interest forces that defeated or drastically changed some proposals in Washington also operated in state capitals. In fact, there were even more organized interests, proportionately, to overcome at the state level than at the national level in order to achieve health care reform. Yet significant state-level reforms were achieved in two of our three policy areas, and progress was made in the third, while the reforms stalled and faltered at the national level.

In chapter 2 we utilized the ESA model to hypothesize that the density and diversity of health interest communities in the states would influence their adoption of new health care policies and their stringency of regulation. In particular, we were interested in influence of communities of health interests representing policy advocates and opponents, as well as the overall density of the interest systems in the states. Our findings reveal differential effects of these interest communities on reform outcomes. In the case of pharmacy assistance programs, neither interest advocates nor opponents had an impact on the likelihood of policy adoption. However, advocates were positively associated with successful efforts to expand and increase the generosity of pharmacy programs once they were enacted. In the case of managed care reforms, we observed a significant influence of communities of both health interest advocates and opponents of reform, with advocates triumphing in the contagion of regulatory adoptions that swept the states. We also observed a crowding effect, whereby states with more crowded health interest communities were less likely to achieve reforms. Finally, in the case of universal coverage, we again observed a significant influence of communities of both health interest advocates and opponents, but no crowding effect. We speculate that the standoff among organized interests prevented state policymakers from jumping on a universal coverage bandwagon; rather, the adoption graph shows a couple of smaller spikes, though consideration of the policy was continuous among states up to the enactment of the ACA in 2010.

Our findings of a differential influence of health interest organizations across our three policies can be summarized in terms of the traits of each reform effort. Our three reforms—pharmaceutical assistance programs, managed care reforms, and universal coverage policies—represent both regulatory and expenditure programs, as well as relatively small and large changes from the status quo. Figure 6.1 arranges the three reforms along these dimensions and summarizes the impact of health interest organizations in each case. The case of pharmacy assistance adoption represents an expenditure policy with little divergence from existing policy models. In this case, we found little evidence that the density of health interests and both their diversity and that of the overall interest system had any independent impact on the likelihood of a state adopting a prescription drug program. However, as the policy moved into an arena more akin to regulation, organized interests played a significant role when it came time for fine-tuning eligibility and other criteria of generosity and revision of the prescription drug programs. Program expansion occurred in states having a high proportion of drug interests, presumably because they desired more customers who could afford to purchase their products. Also, such states were characterized by having proportionately more AARP members and fewer health finance interests. Generosity of programs was advanced by having fewer health interests lobbying overall and by having relatively more advocacy interests.

Managed care reforms represent regulatory policies with a clear divergence from the status quo. In this case, our results showed a consistent and significant impact of health interest organizations on resulting reforms. Furthermore, we found that the more health care organizations registered to lobby, proportionately, the fewer regulations enacted and the less stringent are those that do pass. Similarly, where health political action committees contribute more money proportionately, the stringency of regulations is depressed. Although the general pattern observed was rapid passage of managed care reforms in the states, the findings reveal that states with more crowded health interest systems had a harder time passing reforms, especially stringent reforms. The strongest advocacy lobby turned out to be the independent medical care providers; they had a clear positive impact on both the number of anti–managed care regulations passed and the teeth in those regulations.

The most consistent effect of interest organization variables was observed in the struggle over universal coverage, which represents an expenditure policy that greatly diverged from the status quo system. In this case we observed liberal advocacy groups making the most difference on the pro side, whereas on the anti side small business groups, tax groups, and insurance companies reduced the promotion of universal coverage. Unlike the case of managed care reforms, neither the number of total registered interests in a state nor health care providers proportionate to the size of the total lobby depressed pursuit of universal coverage. Rather, the effect was just the opposite, leading to more steps along the universal coverage continuum.

Figure 6.1 Summary of Health Interest Organization Effects on State Reforms

	Expenditure programs	**Regulatory change**
Low departure from status quo	Low impact *(SPAP adoption)*	High impact *(SPAP expansion and generosity)*
High departure from status quo	High impact *(Universal coverage)*	Medium impact *(Managed care)*

Source: Constructed by the authors.

By exploiting variation in different types of policies across the fifty states, our data tell a story in which industry interest groups are present and active at the state level, but other types of interest groups are able to overcome their influences and enact reform. We have shown that the composition of the states' interest organization systems, including the balance of advocates and opposition groups and the overall density of the system, matters for reform. Furthermore, as described in the previous section, the impact of interest organizations is tempered by numerous other factors in the political and policy environment. Looking toward future reforms and the rules and regulations that will govern implementation of the ACA, it will be imperative for both policymakers and observers to shift from a singular focus on the influence of an organized opposition to a broader focus on the entire interest group community and the state level context that surrounds it.

The States Implement (or Not) the Affordable Care Act

The ACA assigns states many different roles, of which three stand out as especially critical. One is that states are to set up and run the health insurance exchanges through which private insurers will offer their products to consumers and small businesses. Another is that states will oversee a considerable expansion of the Medicaid program, mostly paid for by the federal government, but still requiring some state match. The Supreme Court modified the leverage or threat the federal government held over the states, leaving only the enhanced match to entice states to participate (100 percent through 2016, then a 90 percent match from 2020 on). A third task is to modify the regulation of the small group and individual insurance markets in light of new federal consumer protections, such as eliminating exclusions for preexisting conditions and excessive rate variations by health status, sex, age, and tobacco use, as well as the provision of more oversight for proposed health insurance rate increases. Each of these areas is a major challenge in and of itself, in terms both of policy and of the politics surrounding it.

We begin with the establishment of the state insurance exchanges, which were a compromise in the ACA bill between supporters and opponents of the public option. The exchanges allow self-employed people, uninsured individuals, and small businesses with fewer than fifty employees to shop for private insurance in new marketplaces that will provide consumers with better information about competing health plans. The cost of such insurance may be subsidized (for those between 100 and 400 percent of the federal poverty level). In concept insurance exchanges appeal to both liberals and conservatives, though the details often differ by ideological orientation. State insurance exchanges are likely to run the gamut from the precursors set up by Massachusetts in 2006 to the radically different model Utah set up in 2008. In the Bay State the state government serves as an active purchaser, soliciting bids from private insurance companies and negotiating prices and benefits in order to secure the best value for state residents (Pear 2010). The Utah Health Exchange, in contrast, organizes the market loosely, allowing consumers to compare a wide variety of health plans sold by any private insurers that wish to participate. Most states will fall somewhere along the continuum from Boston to Salt Lake City in their combination of regulation and competition, perhaps with larger states emulating Massachusetts and smaller states copying Utah; or perhaps liberal states will copy Massachusetts and conservative states will emulate Utah. Or a liberal state could erect its own public option and offer it through its insurance exchange; this could even be a single-payer system, such as Vermont has enacted. States can also partner with neighboring states to offer regional exchanges; such organizations might make sense in the sparsely populated western states. These exchanges are expected to be the source of coverage for 24 million people, including members of Congress (Weil and Scheppach 2010). If a state is unable or unwilling to run its own exchange, the federal government will do so. Thus, the insurance exchanges offer a panoply of options for states, from installing a single-payer health plan system to complete inaction.

The Obama administration made $2 billion available in planning money to help states set up exchanges by the deadline of January 2014 and offered additional funds to seed new nonprofit cooperative health plans that might eventually compete on the insurance exchanges. In addition, the administration made grants toward the establishment of exchanges in most states, and seven states received large grants for information technology infrastructure work (Kaiser State Health Facts 2012c). In September 2010 California became the first state to enact legislation setting up its Health Benefit Exchange, possibly providing a model for other states. California was able to move quickly on the legislation because in 2007 it had attempted a health reform package where a benefit exchange was seriously discussed (Mulholland 2010). Its exchange permits standardization of plans and authorizes the use of selective contracting to leverage purchasing power. By the end of 2012 nineteen states had decided to establish their own exchanges, seven states had plans for partnership exchanges in cooperation with the federal government (Kaiser State Health Facts 2012c), and the twenty-five remaining states had defaulted to federal exchanges. Many Republican governors had waited for the Supreme Court ruling before implementing the exchange; then they decided to wait for the outcome of the November 2012 elections. However, the tasks were far too great for the fourteen-month window that remained, and some leaders will always be opposed. Thus it is not surprising that out of the twenty-five states that chose not to participate and hence have the federal government run their exchanges, twenty-three were controlled by the Republicans.[1]

President Obama and his administration took a flexible and conciliatory position vis-à-vis the states in 2011 with regard to definition of the coverage package. They announced that they would not define a single uniform set of "essential health benefits" that insurers must provide through the exchanges; rather, they would allow each state to select a benchmark plan that was already in operation that offers coverage in the broad categories required under the ACA (Pear 2011). Obama also signaled his support for legislation that would allow states to obtain waivers from the individual mandate as early as 2014, if states can show that their plan expands coverage without driving up the costs of health care. Such legislation was not greeted warmly by Republican leaders, who preferred to kill the ACA, not amend it (Stolberg and Sack 2011).

A second major task confronting states under the ACA is the incorporation of many newly eligible people onto the Medicaid rolls; this process also must be completed by 2014. The law required that Medicaid be extended to all people under sixty-five years of age with income up to 138 percent of the federal poverty level, which would have increased the program's overall enrollment by about 50 percent. However, the Supreme Court's ruling in June 2012 made the expansion optional for states, so no one knows which states will expand their programs and thus how many new people will be added to Medicaid. Again a number of Republican governors said that they would not participate in the expansion of Medicaid or would not decide until after the November 2012 elections (Scott 2012). Although the federal government will pay the lion's share of expenses for the new Medicaid beneficiaries (100 percent at first, tapering off to 90 percent in 2020 and beyond), even 10 percent of the expenses of the 16 million people estimated to be added to the Medicaid rolls is a large sum of money for cash-strapped states (King 2010). The Supreme Court ruled in June 2012 that a state can continue with its current program even if it chooses not to join the expanded Medicaid program. The enrollment and financial effects will vary across states based on coverage levels in 2010; those with low coverage in 2010 will see the greatest reduction in the uninsured, but also the highest proportion paid for by the federal government in the 2014–19 ramp-up period (Holahan and Headen 2010). Enrollment increases will also depend upon the vigor of the states' outreach programs.

The contrasting reactions of Alabama's and New Mexico's Medicaid directors to their prospects illustrate the states' varied responses to this part of national health reform. Even though Alabama has a lot to gain from the new federal law (insuring more than 350,000 new people for only 3.6 percent more spending), its director saw the deal as a fiscal calamity: "They're doing healthcare reform on the backs of the states . . . and at a time like now, it's just impossible. We cannot do it" (quoted by Buntin 2010, 22). In contrast, in New Mexico, another poor state with the nation's second-highest uninsured rate, the Medicaid director saw health reform as bringing an economic boon to the state: "We shouldn't worry about five years from now. . . . We're going to get a tremendous match" (quoted by Buntin 2010, 22). The result will be a second fiscal stimulus that will help jump-start stalled state economies, the director argued. How much of the difference in the Medicaid directors' viewpoints can be attributed to the fact that one served under a Republican governor (Alabama) and one under a Democrat at that time (New Mexico) is impossible to say, but we do know that after the 2010 elections there were even more Republican governors. Thus, it is safe to predict that state reactions to this now optional part of the ACA will be varied and probably more negative than a 90 percent federal match would normally elicit from governors. By March 2013, fourteen governors—all Republicans—had announced that their states would not participate in expanding Medicaid and three other Republican governors said they were leaning the same way (Advisory Board, 2013). Twenty-five states, seventeen led by Democrats and eight led by Republicans, had decided to participate in the new expanded Medicaid program.[1] Two other Democratic governors were leaning toward particpation. Six governors, mostly Republican, were still undecided or unannounced. Thus partisanship, with a few significant exceptions, continues to be played out here.

The third task for states under the ACA is to provide the increased regulation of the individual and small-group insurance markets called for in some of the act's major titles. Most of the federal law's consumer protections will come from the states' enforcement of these new protections on private insurance companies. The first protection was offered to persons with preexisting conditions that normally might be denied coverage or charged prohibitive rates by private insurance companies. The states were to set up insurance plans by July 1, 2010, for such persons; the Department of Health and Human Services (HHS) provided several billion dollars to finance the high-risk pools. If the states chose not to, the federal government set up high-risk pools instead. Twenty-seven states set up their own high-risk insurance plans, whereas twenty-three states elected to have their programs administered by the federal government (King 2011).[2] These insurance programs will operate until 2014, when private insurers will be prohibited from coverage denials on the basis of preexisting conditions. The states that resisted setting up high-risk insurance pools included Georgia, where the insurance commissioner, a Republican candidate for governor, wrote to HHS secretary Kathleen Sebelius that the program will "ultimately become the financial responsibility of Georgians in the form of an unfunded mandate" (quoted by Haberkorn 2010). Louisiana was another state that opted out of setting up its own pool. Its Republican insurance commissioner, an elected official, said that the state's concern was that it would be stuck with the bill: "On the surface, it appears to me to be a no-brainer. . . . We can't afford this" (quoted by Haberkorn 2010). Thus, one of the first steps in enhancing consumer protection did not go smoothly, with only slightly more than half the states stepping up to operate their own plans. Considering that more than thirty states already had their own preexisting insurance pools before ACA went into effect, this is not an impressive number. And the Republican opposition suggests that the road ahead will be bumpy as more Republican governors and legislators took office in 2011.

A second task in insurance regulation that began immediately under the ACA was to involve the states in the process of reviewing rate increases in health plan premiums and their justification. About half the states already give their state insurance department or commission the legal power to approve or disapprove certain types of rate changes. The new federal law offers $250 million to help states strengthen their oversight capacities and furnishes states without rate review programs assistance in starting them. In the latter case state insurance authorities have to ask state legislatures to expand their regulatory authority. Five states—Alaska, Georgia, Iowa, Wyoming, and Minnesota—had not applied for grant funding by the end of August 2010 (NCSL 2010b). In Minnesota's case Republican governor Tim Pawlenty issued an executive order directing his state's government agencies not to participate in any of the discretionary benefits contained in the federal legislation. The same order stipulated that Minnesota would not participate in the expansion of the Medicaid program (Van Denburg 2010). All these decisions were reversed when Democrat Mark Dayton took control of the governor's office in early 2011. He also moved 95,000 poor Minnesotans onto Medicaid rolls, mostly from other state programs offering inferior benefits (Wolfe 2011). In addition, the law requires all health insurance plans to spend at least 80 percent of premium dollars on medical services and mandates plans in the large group market to spend at least 85 percent; otherwise, plans must provide rebates to policyholders. By August 2012 consumers and businesses expected to receive rebates totaling $1.3 billion from insurers that did not spend enough on patient care (Kaiser State Health Facts 2012a). By 2014 federal law requires that there be no rate variation by health status and by gender, and variation by age is permitted only within a ratio of 3 to 1. These are all matters that state insurance regulators will need to enforce; if they do not, then presumably the federal authorities will step in and do the job for them. State insurance regulation will depend upon state administrative capacity, just as we saw in the case of state HMO regulation, and it will depend upon the political will of elected insurance commissioners and the governors who appoint commissioners.

Clearly, in all three of these areas the states have critical roles to play in the implementation of the ACA. Implementation will depend heavily upon the bureaucratic capacity and expertise of state health departments and insurance departments. Many states have established health reform steering committees or councils to coordinate across the various agencies that will need to be involved in the years-long implementation period, from information technology to children and family services to health to insurance. But implementation also depends upon the political will of state legislators and governors (Skocpol 2010), which may be in short supply following the 2010 and 2011 elections. As a result of those elections Republicans held unified party control of the state legislature and the governorship in twenty-two states, whereas the Democrats held such party control in only eleven states. In sixteen states the situation of divided party control obtained, with each party controlling no more than one institution of state government. Nebraska is nonpartisan. Assuming that most state Republican legislative parties and governors are opposed to the ACA, we can predict that in the twenty-two states held solidly by the Republicans, implementation of the ACA will be challenged in a variety of ways, especially financially. And this will only be intensified after the elections of 2012, which brought unified Republican control to twenty-three states, whereas the Democrats increased their hold on state government to fifteen states. The number of divided party control states shrank to eleven; one state is nonpartisan. Thus the Republicans' ability to be recalcitrant federal partners continues.

Indeed, state challenges to the federal law began almost immediately after the ACA was signed into law and continues even after the Supreme Court's decision. On March 23, 2010, the attorneys general of both the Commonwealth of Virginia and the State of Florida filed lawsuits in federal court seeking to overturn health care reform. Florida's suit was joined by twenty-five other states and the National Federation of Independent Business (NCSL 2012); in addition to the state-initiated lawsuits, a variety of other private parties filed lawsuits related to the federal law.[3]

Besides attorneys general, state legislators busied themselves with expressing their displeasure over the ACA. As of February 2012, forty-seven state legislatures had seen bills introduced that would limit, alter, or oppose selected federal reform actions, including the individual and employer mandates, or that would allow people to buy health insurance across state lines; twenty states had enacted such measures by the fall of 2012. Half the states sought to pursue an "Interstate Healthcare Freedom Compact" (NCSL 2012). Again, Virginia was the first state to adopt a statute, on March 20, 2010, with a section titled "Health Insurance Coverage Not Required" (NCSL 2010b). Six other states had followed in Virginia's footsteps by November 2010. In the area of state constitutional amendments, most states used as their model Arizona's text, which preserves "the freedom of all residents of the state to provide for their own health care" (NCSL 2010b). Arizona's amendment also stated that no law or rule could compel any person to participate in any health care system, and that no person should be required to pay penalties or fines for paying directly for lawful health care services. The amendment was enacted by voters on November 2, 2010, in Arizona and Oklahoma but was rejected in Colorado. Various challenges to the ACA were placed before the voters in five states in November 2012; the amendments failed only in Florida. Other states pursued the "nullification" of federal law relating to health care, whereas legislation offered in still other states directed that federal monies should be returned. Thus, well before the individual mandate was to be required in 2014, political actors in many states attempted to create statutory and constitutional barriers to the ACA's enforcement. By late 2012 a fair number had already succeeded in enacting either a statute or state constitutional amendment, despite the Supreme Court's ruling.

Opposition to the ACA came from states that shared one of two characteristics, though they were often intertwined. One source of opposition already noted is Republican state officials. The attorneys general who filed lawsuits were mostly Republicans (Adamy and Perez 2010). Democrats holding the same office have refused to file lawsuits requested by Republican governors, and in other states Democratic governors have denounced suits filed by Republican attorneys general (Jost 2010). Several Republican governors elected in 2010 made antipathy to the ACA a plank in their platforms; for example, Tennessee's governor, Bill Haslam, denounced it as "an intolerable expansion of federal power" (Aizenman 2010). Another notable characteristic is that the challenges often seem to come from states that need federal help the most. For example, of the twenty-seven states that had filed lawsuits against the federal government by the end of 2012, fourteen rank in the top half of the states in proportions of uninsured. In general, these states stand to benefit greatly from the law but nonetheless are fighting it; of course, many of these states also have Republican leadership. Texas is a good example of such a state: It leads the nation in uninsured, 28 percent of its population. Rather than embracing this opportunity to siphon off billions of federal dollars to cover its obligations to poor Texans, Republican governor Rick Perry has vowed to fight "on every front available" against this example of "socialism on American soil" (Sack 2010). Yet at the same time, Texas state agencies continue to move ahead with implementation of the ACA, including applying for federal grant money, and holding legislative sessions to prepare for Texas's eventual cooperation. Thus the rhetoric from the governor's office and the political theater of the attorney general's office are not necessarily matched by what bureaucrats are quietly doing to prepare for the new law's implementation.

However, there was also evidence that some states and federalism experts regard the ACA as a case of cooperative federalism rather than federal coercion. In the Supreme Court's hearing on the expansion of Medicaid, an amicus brief was filed by eleven states, led by Oregon. It said in part: "The ACA does not disturb the states' autonomy and freedom to experiment that has always been a hallmark of the program" (quoted by Harkness 2012, 17).

At the same time as the ACA is being challenged at the state level, the Republicans who took control of the US House of Representatives after the 2010 elections vowed to repeal the act. However, with the US Senate and the White House under Democratic control, that threat seemed mostly symbolic. The House Republicans can use their power over appropriations to strip out some of the funding for the act's implementation, for example, the monies to set up health benefit exchanges when states do not choose to do so. Repeal depended initially upon what happened in the elections of 2012; with the Democrats maintaining control of the White House and increasing their control of the Senate slightly, outright repeal is not going to happen. But the federal government's continued fiscal problems and the national debt could affect the money available for ACA programs and thus its prospects for success.

Back to the Future

If the Republicans gain control of both houses of Congress in November 2014 and refuse to fund the ACA, what will happen to health care reform? Action will return again to the states as federalism repeats a pendulum swing: Interests defeated at one governmental level turn to the other governmental level. What might happen in the states? Until perhaps 2015 the states will be engaged in recovering financially from the current economic recession and the housing market collapse; after that, many unmet needs may come before much health care reform happens. Until Democrats take back many of the state legislatures and governorships they lost in 2010, little progress will likely be seen on universal coverage. Indeed, initial analysis of voting in the 2010 elections showed that not only were Democratic candidates for congressional office penalized by opponents of the ACA, but the health reform penalty even had state-level coattails: Voters opposed to the ACA were also less likely to vote for Democratic governors and attorneys general, controlling for everything else (Konisky and Richardson 2012). So Democrats have their work cut out for them to regain state-level offices and move ahead again on health care reform.

Even some of the universal coverage plans states enacted at the start of this century seem to be in trouble. Maine's Dirigo health plan has been reduced in size and has been on life support since the election of Tea Party favorite Republican Paul LePage, who repeatedly blasted the program during his campaign. The cochair of his transition team pronounced the program "Dirigone," though he said it would be replaced by something else (Mistler 2010). Vermont's Catamount Health program was on somewhat shaky financial ground and needed a bailout of several million dollars from the state legislature in 2010, but it will now be replaced by the single-payer Green Mountain Care championed by Democratic governor Peter Shumlin. Massachusetts's health care plan seems on the safest ground for now, given its popularity with the public. And the public's support is critical for health care reform to be sustained in the long run, because it will always cost money. If Massachusetts can stay the course, then its program can serve as an example for other states to follow, once economic and political realities have changed. Then universal coverage will no longer be an experiment but will be a well-tested and reasonable solution to vexing public problems of cost and access in health care.

However, because Democrats retained control of the presidency and the Senate in November 2012, state reform will take place within the framework of the ACA, which the Supreme Court upheld essential portions of on June 28, 2012. It is worth asking, then, what the implications of our analysis hold for the future of the act, especially in terms of how organized interests will continue to play a role in the public provision and regulation of health care. At the national level, of course, the issue is far from over. President Obama's signature legislative accomplishment certainly was a major focus of the 2012 presidential campaign. In this national play of politics over health care reform, interest groups will continue to play a significant role, perhaps aligned as they were over the initial passage of the ACA. However, it is far from clear if the issue becomes stripping, modifying, or amending portions of the ACA. Insurance companies, for example, have a powerful interest to support a universal mandate and health exchanges if other provisions of the act having to do with coverage limits and prior medical conditions are retained because they stand to gain many new patients. Hospitals have a strong incentive to lobby states to accept the new Medicaid money so that they can fill beds with new patients and offset some of the cuts the ACA makes in the budgets of hospitals. Still, our special attention has been on the interest organizations in state health reform. Given the Supreme Court's decision, and assuming that the heart of the ACA survives past the 2014 elections and potential policy swings accompanying it, organized interests can be expected to be active at the state level on two major issues associated with the implementation of the ACA.

First, the Supreme Court's decision on the ACA declared unconstitutional the portion of the ACA that imposed a severe penalty on states if they do not expand Medicaid coverage. Such an expansion was a major part of the plan for providing health care insurance coverage for lower-income citizens. But following the decision, the penalty on a state for not expanding coverage cannot be a complete cessation of federal Medicaid funds; a state will still receive federal funds for its current Medicaid program. States will, however, still have significant financial incentives to expand such coverage (a 100 percent match in the short term, and a 90 percent match in the long term). Moreover, we think, the politics of interest organizations in the states will strongly encourage states to opt for such expansion, even though half the states opposed the ACA when the Supreme Court considered it. Medicaid expansion was a key part of the act's implementation of universal coverage, which is expected to cover 17 million of the 33 million the ACA was expected to remove from the ranks of the uninsured. Hospitals and pharmaceutical companies in particular will vigorously protect this new market share by intensively lobbying reluctant states. Also on sober second thought, some Republican governors may realize that the enhanced federal Medicaid match is such a good deal that they do not want to leave money on the table. We expect, therefore, that—perhaps with considerable grumbling among opponents of health care reform—a majority of states will eventually expand coverage at the behest of, if not their lower-income citizens, then the powerful interests who stand to benefit from their coverage.

A second way in which organized interests will play a role in continuing debates over health care reform at the state level concerns the implementation of the ACA. The ACA is a complex piece of legislation that requires the states to play a significant role in its implementation. And our findings in chapters 3 and 4 are especially telling on the issue of state implementation. In chapter 4, on the regulation of HMOs, we saw that state capacity matters very much. States with greater administrative capacity adopted more regulations and were perhaps more responsive to public opinion than those with less. We would expect the same to happen with respect to the implementation of the ACA. States will vary in the alacrity of their responses and the fullness of their responsiveness to the intent of the ACA when they adopt implementation legislation. States with more administrative capacity will do a better job than others, with representatives of more specialized interests playing a significant role in the latter in inhibiting a sense of haste and thoroughness in policymaking. Even more telling, we saw in chapter 3 on state pharmaceutical assistance policies, special interests that might be expected to oppose such laws were far more effective in later modifying state pharmaceutical assistance programs after they were passed than they were in stopping their adoption. After the political spotlight on initial adoption is turned off, the devil will have his say in the details of implementation. Again, because much of what the states do to implement the ACA will concern regulatory policy, we should expect organized interests with large financial stakes in how the ACA is actually implemented to play a significant role in shaping whatever the ACA eventually becomes. The health insurance industry can be expected to lobby states to establish exchanges through which they can sell their products to individuals and small businesses, an estimated 16 million people (Jones, Bradley, and Oberlander 2012, 32). In short, the adoption of the ACA in 2010 and its being substantively upheld by the Supreme Court in 2012 leaves plenty of opportunity for organized interests to later influence health care policy at the state level. The play of politics by organized interests over health care reform will be fascinating to watch in the states for many years to come.

Notes

1. More specifically, the branch of state government that made the decision—legislative or executive—was controlled by the Republicans in 2012.

2. Before the passage of the ACA, thirty-four states operated their own high-risk pools covering nearly 200,000 people who were uninsurable.

3. In four states—Arizona, George, Mississippi, and Nevada—the action was initiated at the behest of the governor.

Appendix 2.1: Descriptions of Health Interest Organization Subguilds

Table A2.1 Descriptions of Health Interest Organization Subguilds

Major Subguild	Subtypes	Kinds of organizations	Sample organizations in category
Direct providers of patient care	Hospitals and medical centers	Hospitals and health centers; hospital organizations, psychiatric hospitals; hospital districts, parent foundations existing to support hospitals; individual hospitals as well as multihospital corporations	Vanderbilt University Medical Center; Alexian Brothers Medical Center; Arkansas Baptist Hospital
	Nursing homes and extended care	Nursing homes; adult care providers; hospices; home care; residential assisted living; long-term care; rehabilitation hospitals, adult day services	Hebrew Home for the Aged at Riverdale; Georgia Nursing Homes; Alive Hospice; Assisted Living Centers of Georgia; Magee Rehabilitation Hospital
	Primary care / doctors' offices, clinics	Clinics, group and individual practices	Austin Regional Clinic; Illinois Primary Health Care Group; North Texas Specialty Physicians; Pennhurst Medical Group
	Treatment facilities	Drug abuse treatment centers; mental health clinics; foot clinics; ambulatory care centers, community cancer centers	Accident and Injury Pain Centers; New Jersey Mental Health Facilities; Sioux Falls Foot Surgical Center

Table A2.1 Descriptions of Health Interest Organization Subguilds

Major Subguild	Subtypes	Kinds of organizations	Sample organizations in category
	Other facilities	Those not concerned with direct treatment: free standing labs; eye banks; blood banks; clinical laboratories; imaging centers	Community Bio-Resources, Inc.; Central Ohio Lions Eye Bank; Neo Gen Screening Inc.; Pathology Medical Laboratories; Total Renal Care, Inc.
	Other health service providers	Associations of occupational therapists; chiropractors; acupuncture; substance abuse; midwives; dieticians; dental hygienists; physician's assistants; respiratory care; veterinarians; school nurses	American Massage Therapy Association; Veterinary Medical Association; Iowa Association of Marriage & Family Therapists; Oregon Association of Naturopathic Physicians
	Managed care plans and HMOs	Managed care plans and HMOs; HMO associations; behavioral managed care; managed care firms subcontracted to run state health programs; disease management firms; correctional health services	Magellan Health Services, Inc.; PacifiCare Health Systems, Inc.; Association of Connecticut HMOs; Charter Behavioral Health Systems
Drugs and health products	Pharmaceuticals	Pharmaceutical manufacturers; pharmacies; pharmacist associations; pharmacy boards; biotechnology firms	American Home Products Corp.; Knoll Pharmaceutical Co.; National Wholesale Druggists Association; Biotechnology Association of Maine
	Health products	Medical imaging, medical supplies; medical device manufacturers; medical disposal; optometric supplies, mobile exam services (dialysis machines, kidney stone crushers, infusion); dietary supplements and over-the-counter meds	Physiome Sciences; American Mobile Surgical Services, Inc.; Association of Diagnostic Imaging Companies; Medical Equipment Dealers Association

Table A2.1 *(continued)*

Major Subguild	Subtypes	Kinds of organizations	Sample organizations in category
Health finance	Health plans	Health plans; health care benefits companies; health plan organizations; dental plans	Blue Cross and Blue Shield; Anthem Inc.; California Association of Small Employer Health Plans; Delta Dental Insurance Co.
	Business services	Consulting; compliance; billing; software; transcripts; audits; staffing; pharmacy benefits managers; third-party administrators; physician practice management services	Automated Health Systems, Inc.; Health Management Systems Inc.; RealMed Corporation; Utah Health Information Network
	Employer health coalitions	Employer-led purchasing plans, group purchasing pools, employer coalitions among related health causes	Employer Alliance for Affordable Health Care; Montana Association of Health Care Purchasers; Texas Business Group on Health
	Insurance	Underwriters, health insurance firms, medical malpractice liability	Health Insurance Association of America; NC Association of Health Underwriters
Local government health agencies	Government	Local public health agencies, licensing boards; state-sponsored health districts or review organizations; quality improvement organizations	Board of Dental Examiners; California Association of Regional Poison Centers; Palm Beach County Health Care District
	Emergency medical services (EMS) and ambulance services	EMS, health transportation firms	Arrowhead EMS Association; EMS Association of Texas; Lifeline Ambulance Service Inc.
Health advocacy	Advocacy	Advocacy groups: those promoting or advocating some cause, with minimal, largely unstructured, or no treatment (if focused around a specific center or facility, coded as treatment facility)	March of Dimes; Maine Alzheimer's Association; AIDS Foundation of Chicago; Area Agencies on Aging; Texas Rural Health Association

Table A2.1 Descriptions of Health Interest Organization Subguilds

Major Subguild	Subtypes	Kinds of organizations	Sample organizations in category
Health professionals and education centers	Health professionals	Associations of those billable and payable by insurance: medical associations; doctors; nurses; dentists; radiologists; ophthalmologists; psychiatrists; psychologists; radiologists	NE Academy of Eye Physicians and Surgeons; American College of OB/GYNs; Massachusetts Podiatric Medical Society
	Education	Health education; medical schools; training and credentialing organizations; biomedical research unconnected to pharmaceutical applications	Alice Aycock Poe Health Education; Georgia Federation of Professional Health Educators; Medical College of Wisconsin

Source: Constructed by the authors.

Appendix 2.2: States Ranked by Health Interest Group Density

Table A2.2 States Ranked by Health Interest Group Density

State	Health Interest Group Density Rank (1 = Low, 50 = High)			
	1990	1997	1998	1999
Alabama	18	15	12	19
Alaska	3	4	4	4
Arizona	31	35	31	36
Arkansas	4	9	10	10
California	47	47	48	48
Colorado	36	26	32	23
Connecticut	34	36	37	35
Delaware	6	3	6	5
Florida	50	50	50	50
Georgia	42	37	28	33
Hawaii	2	1	3	3
Idaho	7	7	5	7
Illinois	40	48	49	47
Indiana	23	27	24	27
Iowa	33	22	22	18
Kansas	26	29	27	29
Kentucky	20	23	25	25
Louisiana	22	25	23	38
Maine	19	16	9	15
Maryland	37	33	38	40
Massachusetts	46	40	46	42

Table A2.2 States' Ranks on Health Interest Group Density

State	Health Interest Group Density Rank (1 = Low, 50 = High)			
	1990	1997	1998	1999
Michigan	49	42	39	41
Minnesota	43	39	36	37
Mississippi	1	13	14	16
Missouri	24	45	43	43
Montana	15	17	17	14
Nebraska	17	14	15	9
Nevada	35	28	26	31
New Hampshire	8	8	13	13
New Jersey	38	38	42	45
New Mexico	25	21	20	26
New York	48	44	45	46
North Carolina	28	24	30	24
North Dakota	16	20	1	2
Ohio	45	43	41	44
Oklahoma	21	30	35	30
Oregon	32	19	18	21
Pennsylvania	44	46	44	39
Rhode Island	11	6	7	11
South Carolina	12	18	19	22
South Dakota	13	5	8	6
Tennessee	29	32	33	34
Texas	41	49	47	49
Utah	10	11	16	17
Vermont	14	12	11	8
Virginia	27	41	40	20
Washington	39	34	34	32
West Virginia	9	10	21	12
Wisconsin	30	31	29	28
Wyoming	5	2	2	1

Source: Calculated by the authors.

Appendix 2.3: Density by Subguild, Raw Numbers in 1998

Table A2.3 Density by Subguild, Raw Numbers in 1998

State	Drugs and Health Products	Health Care Advocacy	Health Finance	Health Professional Assoc. & Education	Local Government Health	Direct Patient Care
Alabama	17	5	3	8	10	31
Alaska	4	4	2	5	0	13
Arizona	20	18	12	17	6	51
Arkansas	10	3	7	9	4	23
California	53	28	22	37	9	125
Colorado	18	9	10	33	3	45
Connecticut	25	10	7	38	9	67
Delaware	15	6	3	6	0	13
Florida	39	34	19	38	10	207
Georgia	23	13	2	22	3	50
Hawaii	9	1	3	5	0	12
Idaho	10	1	4	8	0	14
Illinois	33	20	13	25	6	165
Indiana	22	6	6	21	0	34
Iowa	10	11	4	15	5	32
Kansas	24	12	8	14	3	45
Kentucky	24	8	5	13	1	45
Louisiana	23	4	7	11	2	47
Maine	7	5	6	8	0	24
Maryland	24	17	13	31	4	78
Massachusetts	44	20	15	22	11	134
Michigan	31	19	9	22	5	89
Minnesota	30	24	11	23	10	56
Mississippi	7	1	5	9	1	20
Missouri	42	17	18	18	12	100

Table A2.3 Density by Subguild, Raw Numbers in 1998

State	Drugs and Health Products	Health Care Advocacy	Health Finance	Health Professional Assoc. & Education	Local Government Health	Direct Patient Care
Montana	11	4	6	17	2	23
Nebraska	16	6	2	13	2	28
Nevada	13	5	10	12	3	53
New Hampshire	9	3	8	9	0	30
New Jersey	34	10	16	22	5	105
New Mexico	19	8	7	16	1	31
New York	36	29	17	29	7	110
North Carolina	26	16	9	20	2	48
North Dakota	5	2	2	4	0	7
Ohio	31	17	18	31	7	84
Oklahoma	24	16	8	22	2	67
Oregon	18	6	5	17	2	25
Pennsylvania	40	16	17	29	2	120
Rhode Island	10	7	5	9	0	14
South Carolina	17	7	5	18	2	30
South Dakota	9	5	3	13	0	18
Tennessee	22	13	10	16	4	61
Texas	45	10	35	30	3	134
Utah	17	6	11	12	1	23
Vermont	13	9	3	10	2	25
Virginia	41	23	14	25	3	78
Washington	29	11	10	23	3	62
West Virginia	20	5	7	15	3	38
Wisconsin	19	11	18	19	3	44
Wyoming	3	1	3	4	0	9

Source: Calculated by the authors.

Appendix 2.4: Data Source for Political Action Committees

The data on contributions to 1998 state electoral campaigns were provided by the National Institute on Money in State Politics.[1] Several caveats about these data must be noted. First, though the National Institute at times refers to the organizations it lists as political action committees (PACs), this name is not really appropriate in the sense in which it is used in the data on national PACs. That is, not all states legally define PACs or, even when they do, define them in the same manner. Indeed, the entities in the National Institute's database include legally defined PACs, other groups that probably are PACs (e.g., the Alabama Dental Association), and individual businesses. Although, for simple convenience, we continue to refer to these entities as PACs, they should more appropriately be interpreted as "nonindividual, nonparty" contributors to political campaigns, as the National Institute more formally calls them. Second, the raw data generously provided by the National Institute through special data requests still required considerable cleaning before they were usable. That is, the state lists included large numbers of individual contributors and duplication of contributors. Recoding to eliminate these cases reduced the initial list of 222,592 PACs to 162,352 PACs. Thus, our experience should serve as a cautionary tale to researchers who are using the National Institute's data without further refinement. Third, we removed party leadership PACs from our data set on the grounds that theoretically they are not interest groups, the subject of our study. And fourth, 1998 data were not available for eight states, usually due to their electoral calendars. In these cases, we used the next available election year, which was either 1999 or 2000.[2] Nonetheless, as a result of all of these adjustments, we believe that our data set contains the best data on state health PACs in existence. And it matches up at the organizational level with our lobbying data set using 1998 lobby registrations; thus we capture both forms of organized interest activity for a single year.

Entities on both lists (whether PACs or lobby registrations) were individually identified as having health interests using the coding rules employed by

Lowery and Gray (2007). The health PACs and lobby registrants were further coded by several subtypes of health interests using the same coding rules. Finally, the cleansed list of PACs was matched with the lobby registration data at the individual organization level to identify whether an organization was registered to lobby, contributed to political campaigns, or both. For the latter two categories, we also measured the size of the financial contribution the organization made to political campaigns for legislative offices, gubernatorial offices, all statewide offices, and judicial candidates.

Notes

1. National Institute on Money in State Politics, "Political Giving Database," www.followthemoney.org/index.phtml.

2. The exceptions are as follows: Arkansas (2000), Delaware (2000), Mississippi (1999), Nebraska (2000), New Jersey (1999), Oklahoma (2000), South Dakota (2000), and Virginia (1999).

Appendix 3.1: List of Data Sources

AARP membership data, annual: AARP Public Policy Institute, *Reforming the Health Care System: State Profiles* (Washington, DC: AARP Public Policy Institute, 2001). Data for 1990–98 were made available by Ethan Bernick.

Date of first adoption and later adoptions: National Conference of State Legislatures, "State Pharmaceutical Assistance Programs, 2004 Edition" (2004), www.ncsl.org/programs/health/drugaid.htm.

Extent of coverage: National Conference of State Legislatures, "State Pharmaceutical Assistance Programs, 2004 Edition" (2004), www.ncsl .org/programs/health/drugaid.htm.

HMO penetration: US Bureau of the Census, *Statistical Abstract of the United States, 2000* (Washington, DC: US Government Printing Office, 2000); Kathleen O'Leary Morgan, Scott Morgan, and Neal Quitno, eds., *Health Care State Rankings, 1994* (Lawrence, KS: Morgan Quitno Press, 1994); Kathleen O'Leary Morgan, Scott Morgan, and Neal Quitno, eds., *Health Care State Rankings, 1995* (Lawrence, KS: Morgan Quitno Press, 1995); Kathleen O'Leary Morgan, Scott Morgan, and Neal Quitno, eds., *Health Care State Rankings, 1996* (Lawrence, KS: Morgan Quitno Press, 1996); Kathleen O'Leary Morgan and Scott Morgan, eds., *Health Care State Rankings, 2001* (Lawrence, KS: Morgan Quitno Press, 2001); Kendra Hovey and Harold Hovey, *CQ's State Fact Finder 1998* (Washington, DC: CQ Press, 1998); Kendra Hovey and Harold Hovey, *CQ's State Fact Finder 1999* (Washington, DC: CQ Press, 1999); Kendra Hovey and Harold Hovey, *CQ's State Fact Finder 2000* (Washington, DC: CQ Press, 2000); Kendra Hovey and Harold Hovey, *CQ's State Fact Finder 2001* (Washington, DC: CQ Press, 2001).

Income eligibility: National Conference of State Legislatures, "State Pharmaceutical Assistance Programs, 2004 Edition" (2004), www.ncsl .org/programs/health/drugaid.htm; National Governors Association, "State Pharmaceutical Assistance Programs, December 17, 2001," www .nga.org/cda/files/STATEPHARM.pdf; US General Accounting Office, "State Pharmacy Programs: Assistance Designed to Target Coverage and

Stretch Budgets: Report to Congressional Requesters," September 2000, GAO/HEHS-00-162; S. Crystal, T. Trail, K. Fox, and J. Cantor, *Enrolling Eligible Persons in Pharmacy Assistance Programs: How States Do It* (New York: Commonwealth Fund, 2003).

Neighbor adoptions: The proportion of neighboring states, lagged by one year, that had already adopted a drug subsidy policy in previous years. Neighboring states are defined by Berry and Berry (1990, 412).

Newspaper stories: an annual count of the terms "senior citizens" and "prescription drugs" in newspaper headlines or lead paragraphs of national newspapers included in the Lexis/Nexis database, lagged by one year.

Opinion liberalism: "Erikson, Wright and McIver, CBS / *New York Times* National Polls, Ideological Identification, 1977–1999," http://mypage .iu.edu/~wright1/.

Per capita gross state product: US Bureau of Economic Affairs, http://www .bea.gov/bea/regional/gsp/.

Per capita prescription drug spending: Kathleen O'Leary Morgan, Scott Morgan, and Neal Quitno, eds., *Health Care State Rankings, 1994* (Lawrence, KS: Morgan Quitno Press, 1994); Kathleen O'Leary Morgan, Scott Morgan, and Neal Quitno, eds., *Health Care State Rankings, 1995* (Lawrence, KS: Morgan Quitno Press, 1995); Kathleen O'Leary Morgan, Scott Morgan, and Neal Quitno, eds., *Health Care State Rankings, 1996* (Lawrence, KS: Morgan Quitno Press, 1996); Kathleen O'Leary Morgan and Scott Morgan, eds., *Health Care State Rankings, 2001* (Lawrence, KS: Morgan Quitno Press, 2001).

Percent change in state revenue: the percentage change (increase or decrease) in state revenue from the previous year.

Percentage of the population sixty-five years and older: US Bureau of the Census, Population Estimates, http://eire.census.gov/popest/estimates .php.

Program limits: National Conference of State Legislatures, "State Pharmaceutical Assistance Programs, 2004 Edition," www.ncsl.org/ programs/health/drugaid.htm; National Governors Association, "State Pharmaceutical Assistance Programs, December 17, 2001," www.nga.org/ cda/files/STATEPHARM.pdf.

Ranney Index, folded: We use the average folded Ranney Index for several periods. The data for the years 1990–94 use the average folded Ranney Index for 1989–94. The data years 1995–98 use the average index for 1995–98. The data years 1999–2001 use the average index from 1999 to 2003. The data were extracted from Virginia Gray and Russell Hanson, eds., *Politics in the American States: A Comparative Analysis*, 6th–8th editions (Washington, DC: CQ Press).

State party control: Council of State Governments, *The Book of the States, 1990–1991* (Lexington, KY: Council of State Governments, 1990); Council of State Governments, *The Book of the States, 1992–1993* (Lexington, KY: Council of State Governments, 1992); and Council of State Governments, *The Book of the States, 1994–1995* (Lexington, KY: Council of State Governments, 1994).

Appendix 3.2: Estimation of Annual Interest Group Measures Using the ESA Model

As seen in table A3.2, 1990 and 1999 numbers of total health, pharmacy, advocacy, and health finance registrations were regressed on gross state product (GSP) and its square to tap the linear and density-dependent elements of the supply of organized interests as well as on a 1999 indicator and its interactions with GSP and its square. The 1999 indicator and its interactions assess how the intercepts and GSP and GSP-squared estimates changed from 1990 to 1999.[1] These estimates were combined with annual data on GSP to generate annual estimates of the total number of health registrations and the proportions arising from our three subguilds.

Table A3.2 ESA Model of Lobby Registrations, 1990 and 1999

Independent Variables	Dependent Variables				
	Pharmacy Registrations	Health Advocacy Registrations	Health Finance Registrations	All Health Registrations	% For-Profit Registrations
GSP	5.714***	7.269***	2.986***	59.567**	0.765
	1.214	2.310	0.946	15.896	0.470
GSP^2	−3.226**	−5.437*	−1.203	−44.881**	−1.836
	1.502	2.752	1.154	19.432	1.522
1999 Dummy	0.863***	0.515***	0.092	3.258*	−0.080
	0.163	0.111	0.112	1.016	0.142
1990 x GSP	−0.100	−0.414**	−0.036	−2.006	0.092
	0.130	0.169	0.107	1.202	0.121
1990 x GSP^2	0.082**	0.489**	−0.008	2.670*	−0.020
	0.136	0.233	0.122	1.576	0.149
Constant	2.923	1.509	3.803	25.570	71.769
R-Square	0.582	0.494	0.299	0.530	0.085
N	100	100	100	100	100

***$p < 0.01$, **$p < 0.05$, *$p < 0.10$, two-tailed tests, robust standard errors clustered on state.
Source: Reprinted with permission from Gray, Lowery, and Godwin (2007b).

Note

1. We do not discuss these models in detail except to note that they work as well as single-year ESA models, but indicate that pharmacy and total health registrations became somewhat less density dependent over the 1990s. It is worth mentioning, however, that when the proportion of for-profit registrations was examined using the same models, as seen in the last column of table A3.2, the results were extremely weak. In short, this proportion has not changed much over almost three decades, which justifies our sole use of this static measure of the opposition to SPAPs, as discussed above.

Appendix 4.1: Data Sources of Dependent Variables

Data on liability regulations were obtained from the National Council of State Legislatures, "Managed Care Insurer Liability," www.ncsl.org/programs/health/liable.htm.

Data on external review requirements were obtained from Health Policy Tracking Service, Issue Brief, "Consumer Grievance Procedures: Internal and Independent Appeals" (Year End Report, 2003).

Data on ombudsman and report card laws are from National Council of State Legislatures, "Managed Care Insurer State Laws for Ombudsman, Report Cards and Provider Profiles," www.ncsl.org/programs/health/hmorep2.htm.

Data on internal reviews are from Health Policy Tracking Service, Issue Brief, "Consumer Grievance Procedures: 'Internal and Independent Appeals'" (Year End Report, 2003).

Data on any willing provider laws are from Health Policy Tracking Service, Issue Brief, "Any Willing Provider" (Year End Report, 2003).

Data on bans on provider financial incentives are from Health Policy Tracking Service, Issue Brief, "Bans on Financial Incentives" (Year End Report, 2003), December 31, 2003.

Data on continuity of care rules were obtained from Health Policy Tracking Service, Issue Brief, "Continuity of Care" (Year End Report, 2003), December 31, 2003.

Data on standing referral laws are from the Kaiser Family Foundation, "Patients' Rights: Standing Referrals for Ongoing Care with a Specialist, 2003," available at statehealthfacts.org.

Data on access to obstetrician-gynecologists are from Kaiser Family Foundation, "State Mandated Benefits: Direct Access to OB/GYNS, 2003," available at statehealthfacts.org.

Data on gag bans are from Health Policy Tracking Service, Issue Brief, "Bans on Gag Clauses" (Year End Report, 2003), December 31, 2003.

Appendix 4.2: Managed Care Regulation Descriptive Statistics

Table A4.2 Managed Care Regulation Descriptive Statistics

Variable	Mean	Standard Deviation
DV: Number of provisions	7.30	2.24
DV: Stringency of provisions	-0.01	5.19
DV: Weighted number of provisions	14.74	4.72
DV: Weighted stringency of provisions	-0.02	10.78
Health proportion of all contributions	0.04	0.05
Folded Ranney index	0.87	0.09
Opinion liberalism	-0.14	0.10
HMO penetration	21.80	13.32
Malpractice suit rate	21.44	8.27
Administrative capacity	3.04	0.61
Per capita GSP	0.03	0.005
Health advocacy percentage	10.57	4.80
Independent care provider percentage	1.43	1.18
HMO percentage	7.74	3.39
Health business percentage	7.83	2.95
Law percentage of all registrations	2.16	0.96
Health percentage of all registrations	16.87	7.06

Table A4.2 (*continued*)

Variable		Mean	Standard Deviation
		Frequency	Percent
Democratic governor	0	27	54
	0.5	10	20
	1	13	26
Democratic legislature	0	16	32
	0.25	3	6
	0.5	9	18
	0.75	3	6
	1	19	38

Source: Calculated by the authors.

Appendix 4.3: Definitions and Sources of Independent Variables

Table A4.3 Definitions and Sources of Independent Variables

Variables	Definitions
Political variables	
Party competition	Average of 1997 and 1999 folded Ranney indices
Opinion liberalism	Erikson, Wright, and McIver, http://mypage .iu.edu/'~wright1/
Democratic Party control	Average of 1997 and 1999 values of Democratic Party control of State House, Senate, and governorship, each coded 1.
Need variables	
HMO penetration	Average of 1997 and 1999 proportion of populations in HMOs
Malpractice suit rate	No. of physician malpractice payments, annualized rate per 1,000 practitioners, September 1, 1990– December 31, 1996, www.npdb-hipdb.com/pubs/ stats/1996_NPDB_Annual_.Report.pdf
Capacity variables	
Administrative capacity	Governing.com ranking of administrative capacity of the states, 1999, http://governing.com/ gpp/2001/gp1glanc.htm
State wealth	Average of 1997 and 1999 per capita gross state product
Interest organization variables	
Health advocacy proportion	Average of 1997 and 1999 proportion of all health guild lobby registrations by health advocacy organizations
Independent care provider proportion	Average of 1997 and 1999 proportion of all health guild lobby registrations by independent care provider organizations

Table A4.3 (*continued*)

Variables	Definitions
HMO proportion	Average of 1997 and 1999 proportion of all health guild lobby registrations by health maintenance organizations
Health business proportion	Average of 1997 and 1999 proportion of all health guild lobby registrations by insurance companies or associations, other health plans, and business health coalitions
Law proportion	Average of 1997 and 1999 proportion of all lobby registrations by legal organizations
Health proportion	Average of 1997 and 1999 proportion of all lobby registrations by health organizations
Health PAC proportion	Proportion of all contributions from health sector, 1998, National Institute on Money in State Politics

Source: Reprinted with permission from Gray, Lowery, and Godwin (2007a).

Appendix 5.1: Sources of Dependent Variables

Primary Sources for Universal Health Care Bills

1988–89 bills: Guided Search of Lexis/Nexis Academic Newspaper Database. Key words used in search: "universal health care" or "universal health insurance" or "universal health access." Accessed at http://web.lexis-nexis.com/universe/form/ academic/s_guidednews.html.

1990–91 bills: Search of 50-State Bill Tracking and Bill Full Text Database of Lexis/Nexis State Capital Universe. Key words used: "universal health care" or "universal health coverage" or "universal health insurance" or "universal health access" or "comprehensive health coverage" or "single-payer health care." Accessed at www.lexisnexis.com/academic, by subscription.

1992 bills: Kala Ladenheim, *State Health Care Reform Legislation* (Washington, DC: Congressional Research Service, 1993); Merit Kimball, ed., *Major Health Legislation in the States: '92* (Washington, DC: Intergovernmental Health Policy Project, George Washington University, 1993).

1993 bills: Lisa Atchison, Lisa Bowleg, Donna Folkemer, Dick Hegner, Claire Helf, Tim Henderson, Kala Ladenheim, Helen Leeds, Anne Markus, and Jacqueline Morgan, *Major Health Legislation in the States: 1993* (Washington, DC: Intergovernmental Health Policy Project, 1994).

1994 bills: Lisa Atchison, Lisa Bowleg, Donna Folkemer, Richard Hegner, Claire Helf, Tim Henderson, Kala Ladenheim, Helen Leeds, and Anne Markus, *Major Health Legislation in the States: 1994* (Washington, DC: Intergovernmental Health Policy Project, George Washington University, 1994).

1995 bills: Search of 50-State Bill Tracking and Bill Full Text Database of Lexis/Nexis State Capital Universe; Kelly Perez and Barbara Wright, *Health*

Care Legislation 1995 (Denver: National Conference of State Legislatures, 1996).

1996 bills: Search of 50-State Bill Tracking and Bill Full Text Database of Lexis/Nexis State Capital Universe; National Conference of State Legislatures Health Care Program, *Health Care Legislation 1996* (Denver: National Conference of State Legislatures, 1997).

1997 bills: Search of 50-State Bill Tracking and Bill Full Text Database of Lexis/Nexis State Capital Universe; Laura Tobler, Martha King, Rhonda Gonzalez, et al., *Health Care Legislation 1997* (Denver: National Conference of State Legislatures, 1998).

1998–2002 bills: National Conference of State Legislatures, "Status Report: Universal Health Care State Legislation," March 2002, personal communication from Richard Cauchi, National Conference of State Legislatures.

2003–4 bills: National Conference of State Legislatures, "Universal Health Care: 2005 Legislation," www.ncsl.org/default.aspx?tabid=13876.

Supplementary Sources

1997–2004: Search of Health Policy Tracking Service Database in "Finance Category"; "Access to Health Insurance Subcategory," accessed at www.hpts.org, by subscription.

2003: State Coverage Initiatives, "State Coverage Matrix," accessed at www.statecoverage.net.

1992–2003: Search of American Political Network's "American Health Line," available through Lexis/Nexis State Capital Universe, accessed at www.lexisnexis.com/academic, by subscription.

1993–2003: Search of StateNet's "State Capitols Report," available through Lexis/Nexis State Capital Universe, accessed at www.lexisnexis.com/academic, by subscription.

Appendix 5.2:
Sources of Independent Variables

Gross state product: US Bureau of Economic Affairs, www.bea.doc.gov/bea/regional/gsp/.

HMO penetration: Group Health Association of America, *Patterns in HMO Enrollment: GHAA 1991 Edition* (Washington, DC: Research and Analysis Department, Group Health Association of America, 1991); US Bureau of the Census, *Statistical Abstract of the United States, 2000* (Washington, DC: US Government Printing Office, 2000); Kathleen O'Leary Morgan, Scott Morgan, and Neal Quitno, eds., *Health Care State Rankings, 1993* (Lawrence, KS: Morgan Quitno Press, 1993); Kathleen O'Leary Morgan, Scott Morgan, and Neal Quitno, eds., *Health Care State Rankings, 1994* (Lawrence, KS: Morgan Quitno Press, 1994); Kathleen O'Leary Morgan, Scott Morgan, and Neal Quitno, eds., *Health Care State Rankings, 1995* (Lawrence, KS: Morgan Quitno Press, 1995); Kathleen O'Leary Morgan, Scott Morgan, and Neal Quitno, eds., *Health Care State Rankings, 1996* (Lawrence, KS: Morgan Quitno Press, 1996); Kathleen O'Leary Morgan and Scott Morgan, eds., *Health Care State Rankings, 1997* (Lawrence, KS: Morgan Quitno Press, 1997); Kathleen O'Leary Morgan, Scott Morgan, and Mark Uhlig, eds., *Health Care State Rankings, 1998* (Lawrence, KS: Morgan Quitno Press, 1998); Kathleen O'Leary Morgan and Scott Morgan, eds., *Health Care State Rankings, 1999* (Lawrence, KS: Morgan Quitno Press, 1999); Kathleen O'Leary Morgan and Scott Morgan, eds., *Health Care State Rankings, 2000* (Lawrence, KS: Morgan Quitno Press, 2000); Kathleen O'Leary Morgan and Scott Morgan, eds., *Health Care State Rankings, 2001* (Lawrence, KS: Morgan Quitno Press, 2001); Kathleen O'Leary Morgan and Scott Morgan, eds., *Health Care State Rankings, 2002* (Lawrence, KS: Morgan Quitno Press, 2002); Kathleen O'Leary Morgan and Scott Morgan, eds., *Health Care State Rankings, 2003* (Lawrence, KS: Morgan Quitno Press, 2003); US Bureau of the Census,

Statistical Abstract of the United States, 2004–2005 (Washington, DC: US Government Printing Office, 2005).

Party control of government (lower house, upper house, and governor): Council of State Governments, *The Book of the States, 1980–1981* (Lexington, KY: Council of State Governments, 1980); Council of State Governments, *The Book of the States, 1982–1983* (Lexington, KY: Council of State Governments, 1982); Council of State Governments, *The Book of the States, 1984–1985* (Lexington, KY: Council of State Governments, 1984); Council of State Governments, *The Book of the States, 1986–1987* (Lexington, KY: Council of State Governments, 1986); Council of State Governments, *The Book of the States, 1988–1989* (Lexington, KY: Council of State Governments, 1988); Council of State Governments, *The Book of the States, 1990–1991* (Lexington, KY: Council of State Governments, 1990); Council of State Governments, *The Book of the States, 1992–1993* (Lexington, KY: Council of State Governments, 1992); Council of State Governments, *The Book of the States, 1994-1995* (Lexington, KY: Council of State Governments, 1994) Council of State Governments, *The Book of the States, 1996–1997* (Lexington, KY: Council of State Governments, 1996); Council of State Governments, *The Book of the States, 1998–1999* (Lexington, KY: Council of State Governments, 1998); Council of State Governments, *The Book of the States, 2000–2001* (Lexington, KY: Council of State Governments, 2000); Council of State Governments, *The Book of the States, 2002* (Lexington, KY: Council of State Governments, 2002); Council of State Governments, *The Book of the States, 2003* (Lexington, KY: Council of State Governments, 2003); Council of State Governments, *The Book of the States, 2004* (Lexington, KY: Council of State Governments, 2004).

Personal health care expenditures, percent growth in: Centers for Medicare and Medicaid Services, Office of the Actuary, National Health Statistics Group, www.cms.hhs.gov/statistics/nhe/state-estimates-provider/2000/states.pdf.

Population of state: US Bureau of Economic Affairs, www.bea.doc.gov/bea/regional/spi/.

Prescription drug spending, percent growth in: Centers for Medicare and Medicaid Services, Office of the Actuary, State Health Accounts, www.cms.hhs.gov/statistics/nhe/state-estimates-provider/2000/states.pdf, years 1980–2000; Kaiser Foundation, personal communication from Hannah Yang Moore, years 2001, 2002; Kaiser Foundation, www.statehealthfacts.kff.org, year 2003.

Public opinion liberalism: "Erikson, Wright and McIver, CBS/*New York Times* National Polls, Ideological Identification, 1976–2003," http://mypage .iu.edu/~wright1/.

Ranney Index, folded: We use the average folded Ranney Index for several periods. The data years 1990–94 use the average folded Ranney Index for 1989–94. The data years 1995–98 use the average index for 1995–98. The data years 1999–2001 use the average index for 1999–2003. The data were extracted from Virginia Gray and Russell Hanson, eds., *Politics in the American States: A Comparative Analysis*, 6th–8th editions (Washington, DC: CQ Press).

Total revenue of states: US Bureau of the Census, *Statistical Abstract of the United States, 1989* (Washington, DC: US Government Printing Office, 1989); US Bureau of the Census, *Statistical Abstract of the United States, 1990* (Washington, DC: US Government Printing Office, 1990); US Bureau of the Census, *Statistical Abstract of the United States, 1991* (Washington, DC: US Government Printing Office, 1991); US Bureau of the Census, *Statistical Abstract of the United States, 1992* (Washington, DC: US Government Printing Office, 1992); US Bureau of the Census, *Statistical Abstract of the United States, 1993* (Washington, DC: US Government Printing Office, 1993); US Bureau of the Census, *Statistical Abstract of the United States, 1994* (Washington, DC: US Government Printing Office, 1994); US Bureau of the Census, *Statistical Abstract of the United States, 1995* (Washington, DC: US Government Printing Office, 1995); US Bureau of the Census, *Statistical Abstract of the United States, 1996* (Washington, DC: US Government Printing Office, 1996); US Bureau of the Census, *Statistical Abstract of the United States, 1997* (Washington, DC: US Government Printing Office, 1997); US Bureau of the Census, *Statistical Abstract of the United States, 1998* (Washington, DC: US Government Printing Office, 1998); US Bureau of the Census, *Statistical Abstract of the United States, 1999* (Washington, DC: US Government Printing Office, 1999); US Bureau of the Census, *Statistical Abstract of the United States, 2000* (Washington, DC: US Government Printing Office, 2000); US Bureau of the Census, *Statistical Abstract of the United States, 2001*(Washington, DC: US Government Printing Office, 2001); US Bureau of the Census, *Statistical Abstract of the United States, 2002* (Washington, DC: US Government Printing Office, 2002); US Bureau of the Census, *Statistical Abstract of the United States, 2003* (Washington, DC: US Government Printing Office, 2003); US Bureau of the Census, *Statistical Abstract of the United States, 2004–2005*, online edition at www.census.gov/prod/www/statistical-abstract-04.html.

Uninsured as percentage of population under sixty-five years of age: US Bureau of the Census, Housing and Household Economic Statistics Division, Historical Health Insurance Tables, www.census.gov/hhes/www/hlthins/historic/index.html.

References

AAHP (American Association of Health Plans). 2001. *Health Plan Liability: What You Need to Know.* Available at www.aahp.org.

———. 2002. "Rising Health Care Costs." Available at www.aahp.org.

Abelson, Reed. 2010. "In Health Care Overhaul, Boons for Hospitals and Drug Makers." *New York Times.* March 21. www.nytimes.com/2010/03/22/business/22bizhealth.html?ref=health_care_reform.

Adamy, Janet, and Evan Perez. 2010. "US Fights Challenge to Health Law." *Wall Street Journal,* June 18. http://online.wsj.com/article/SB100014240527487036506045753131308 38206948.html?KEYWORDS=medicaid #printMode.

Advisory Board. 2013. "Daily Briefing: Where Each State Stands on ACA's Medicaid Expansion." March 4. www.advisory.com/Daily-Briefing/2012 /11/09/MedicaidMap.

Aizenman, N. C. 2010. "New GOP Governors Will Affect Health Law." *Washington Post,* November 9. www.washingtonpost.com/wp-dyn/content /article/2010/11/08/AR2010110806367_pf.html.

Allen, Mahally D., Carrie Pettus, and Donald P. Haider-Markel. 2004. "Making the National Local: Specifying the Conditions for National Government Influence on State Policymaking." *State Politics and Policy Quarterly* 4 (Fall): 318–44.

Alliance for Health Reform. 2002. *Sourcebook for Journalists.* www.allhealth .org/sourcebook2002/ch11_tc.html.

American Legislative Exchange Council. 2011. "The State Legislators Guide to Repealing Obamacare." www.alec.org/wp-content/uploads/State_Leg_ Guide_to_Repealing_ObamaCare.pdf

———. 2012. "Health Care Freedom Initiative." www.alec.org/initiatives/ health-care-freedom-initiative/about-alecs-freedom-of-choice-in-health-care-act/.

Arsneault, Shelly. 2000. "Welfare Policy Innovation and Diffusion: Section 1115 Waivers and the Federal System." *State and Local Government Review* 32 (Winter): 49–60.

Balla, Steven J. 2001. "Interstate Professional Associations and the Diffusion of Policy Innovations." *American Politics Research* 29 (May): 221–45.

Barrett, Katherine, and Richard Greene. 1999. "Grading the States, 1999." *Governing*, February. Available at www.governing.com.

Barrilleaux, Charles, and Evan Bernick. 2003. "'Deservingness,' Discretion, and the State Politics of Welfare Spending, 1990–1996." *State Politics and Policy Quarterly* 1:1–18.

Barrilleaux, Charles, and Paul Brace. 2007. "Notes from the Laboratories of Democracy: State Government Enactments of Market- and State-Based Health Insurance Reforms in the 1990s." *Journal of Health Politics, Policy and Law* 32 (August): 655–82.

Barrilleaux, Charles, Paul Brace, and Bruce Dangremond. 1994. "The Sources of State Health Reform." Paper presented at Annual Meeting of American Political Science Association, New York, September.

Barrilleaux, Charles J., and Mark E. Miller. 1988. "The Political Economy of State Medicaid Policy." *American Political Science Review* 82:1089–1107.

Baumgartner, Frank R., Jeffrey M. Berry, Marie Hojnacki, David C. Kimball, and Beth L. Leech. 2009. *Lobbying and Policy Change: Who Wins, Who Loses, and Why.* Chicago: University of Chicago Press.

Baumgartner, Frank R., Virginia Gray, and David Lowery. 2009. "Federal Policy Activity and the Mobilization of State Lobbying Organizations." *Political Research Quarterly* 62 (September): 552–67.

Baumgartner, Frank R., and Bryan D. Jones. 1993. *Agendas and Instability in American Politics.* Chicago: University of Chicago Press.

———. 2009. *Agendas and Instability in American Politics*, 2nd ed. Chicago: University of Chicago Press.

Baumgartner, Frank R., and Bryan D. Jones., eds. 2002. *Policy Dynamics.* Chicago: University of Chicago Press.

Baumgartner, Frank R., and Beth L. Leech. 1996. "Lobbying Disclosure Reports Dataset." http://lobby.la.psu.edu/related.html.

Baumgartner, Frank R., and Jeffery C. Talbert. 1995. "From Setting a National Agenda on Health Care to Making Decisions in Congress." *Journal of Health Politics, Policy and Law* 20 (Summer): 437–45.

Beaussier, Anne-Laure. 2012. "The Patient Protection and Affordable Care Act: The Victory of Unorthodox Lawmaking." *Journal of Health Politics, Policy and Law* 37 (October): 741–78.

Berkman, Michael, and Christopher Reenock. 2004. "Incremental Consolidation and Comprehensive Reorganization of American State Executive Branches." *American Journal of Political Science* 48:796–812.

Bernick, Ethan M., and Nathan Myers. 2008. "Treatment or Placebo: Are State Programs Decreasing the Proportion of Uninsured?" *Political Studies Journal* 36 (3): 367–84.

Berry, Frances Stokes, and William D. Berry. 1990. "State Lottery Adoptions as Policy Innovations: An Event History Analysis." *American Political Science Review* 84:395–415.

———. 1992. "Tax Innovation in the States: Capitalizing on Political Opportunity." *American Journal of Political Science* 36:715–42.

Berry, Jeffrey. 1977. *Lobbying for the People: The Political Behavior of Public Interest Groups*. Princeton, NJ: Princeton University Press.

———. 1999. *The New Liberalism*. Washington, DC: Brookings Institution Press.

Birkland, Thomas A. 2006. *Lessons of Disaster: Policy Change after Catastrophic Events*. Washington, DC: Georgetown University Press.

Bloche, M. Gregg, and David M. Studdert. 2004. "A Quiet Revolution: Law as an Agent of Health System Change." *Health Affairs* 23 (2): 29–42.

Boeckelman, Keith. 1992. "The Influence of States on Federal Policy Adoptions." *Policy Studies Journal* 20 (3): 365–75.

Boehmke, Frederick J., and Richard Witmer. 2004. "Disentangling Diffusion: The Effects of Social Learning and Economic Competition on State Policy Innovation and Expansion." *Political Research Quarterly* 57 (1): 39–51.

Boushey, Graeme. 2010. *Policy Diffusion Dynamics in America*. New York: Cambridge University Press.

———. 2012. "Punctuated Equilibrium Theory and the Diffusion of Innovations." *Policy Studies Journal* 40 (February): 127–46.

Bovbjerg, Randall R. 2003. "Alternative Models of Federalism: Health Insurance Regulation and Patient Protection Laws." In *Federalism and Health Policy*, edited by John Holahan, Alan Weil, and Joshua M. Wiener. Washington, DC: Urban Institute Press.

Brady, David W., and Daniel P. Kessler. 2010. "Why Is Health Reform So Difficult?" *Journal of Health Politics, Policy and Law* 35 (April): 162–75.

Brasher, Holly, David Lowery, and Virginia Gray. 1999. "State Lobby Registration Data: The Anomalous Case of Florida (and Minnesota Too!)." *Legislative Studies Quarterly* 24 (May): 303–14.

Brown, Lawrence D. 2001. "Anticipated Reactions, Uncommon Denominators: The Political Construction of Managed Care Regulation." In *Understanding Health System Change*, edited by Paul B. Ginsburg and Cara S. Lesser. Chicago: Health Administration Press.

————. 2010. "Pedestrian Paths: Why Path-Dependence Theory Leaves Health Policy Analysis Lost in Space." *Journal of Health Politics, Policy and Law* 35 (August): 643–60.

————. 2011. "The Elements of Surprise: How Health Reform Happened." *Journal of Health Politics, Policy and Law* 36 (June): 419–27.

Brown, Lawrence D., and Elizabeth Eagan. 2004. "The Paradoxical Politics of Provider Reempowerment." *Journal of Health Politics, Policy and Law* 29 (6): 1045–71.

Brown, Lawrence D., and Michael S. Sparer. 2001. "Window Shopping: State Health Reform Politics in the 1990s." *Health Affairs* 20:50–68.

Buntin, John. 2010. "Dueling Diagnosis." *Governing*, February, 20–25.

Burstein, Paul, Shawn Bauldry, and Paul Froese. 2005. "Bill Sponsorship and Congressional Support for Policy Proposals, from Introduction to Enactment or Disappearance." *Political Research Quarterly* 58:295–302.

Calmes, Jackie. 2009. "Clinton's Health Defeat Sways Obama's Tactics." *New York Times*, September 6. www.nytimes.com/2009/09/06/health/policy/06lessons.html?_r=1&scp=4&sq=Calmes%20health%20September%202009&st=cse.

Canon, Bradley C., and Lawrence Baum. 1981. "Patterns of Adoption of Tort Law Innovations: An Application of Diffusion Theory to Judicial Doctrines." *American Political Science Review* 75:975–87.

Casalino, Lawrence P. 2004. "Physicians and Corporations: A Corporate Transformation of American Medicine?" *Journal of Health Politics, Policy and Law* 29 (4–5): 869–84.

Cauchi, Richard. 1999. "Managed Care: Where Do We Go from Here?" *State Legislatures*, March, 14–20.

Center for Responsive Politics. 2010. "The Deregistration Dilemma: Are Lobbyists Quitting the Business as Federal Disclosure Rules Tighten?" www.opensecrets.org/news/Deregistrationreport.pdf.

Ching, Donald D. H. 1980. "The Political Planning of a State Health Insurance Program in Hawaii." In *State Innovations in Health*, edited by Richard Merritt and Susan Mertes. Washington, DC: Intergovernmental Health Policy Project/George Washington University.

Crystal, Stephen, Thomas Trail, Kimberley Fox, and Joel Cantor. 2003. "Enrolling Eligible Persons in Pharmacy Assistance Programs: How States Do It." Commonwealth Fund. www.commonwealthfund.org/~/media/Files/Publications/Fund%20Report/2003/Sep/Enrolling%20Eligible%20Persons%20in%20Pharmacy%20Assistance%20Programs%20%20How%20States%20Do%20It/crystal_pharmassistprogs_590%20pdf.pdf.

Davidoff, Amy J., Bruce Stuart, Thomas Shaffer, J. Samantha Shoemaker, Melissa Kim, and Christopher Zacker. 2010. "Lessons Learned: Who Didn't Enroll in Medicare Drug Coverage in 2006, and Why?" *Health Affairs* 29 (June): 1255–63.

Dorf, Michael C. 2009a. "The Constitutionality of Health Insurance Reform, Part I: The Misguided Libertarian Objection." *Findlaw*, October 21. http://writ.news.findlaw.com/dorf/20091021.html.

———. 2009b. "The Constitutionality of Health Insurance Reform, Part II: Congressional Power." *Findlaw*, November 2. http://writ.news.findlaw.com/scripts/printer_friendly.pl?page=/dorf/20091102.html.

Durenberger, David. 2010. "Reason for Optisism: Key Roles for States, Providers, Insurers." *Commonwealth Fund Blog*. www.commonwealthfund.org/Content/Blog/Jul/Reason-for-Optimism.aspx?view=print.

Erikson, Robert S., Gerald C. Wright, and John P. McIver. 1993. *Statehouse Democracy: Public Opinion and Policy in the American States*. Cambridge: Cambridge University Press.

Eshbaugh-Soha, Matthew, and Kenneth Meier. 2008. "Economic and Social Regulation." In *Politics in the American States: A Comparative Analysis*, 9th ed., edited by Virginia Gray and Russell Hanson. Washington, DC: CQ Press.

Esterling, Kevin M. 2009. "Does the Federal Government Learn from the States? Medicaid and the Limits of Expertise in the Intergovernmental Lobby." *Publius: The Journal of Federalism* 39 (1): 1–21.

Farwell, Jackie. 2012. "LePage Plan Would Cut MaineCare Coverage for Families Making More than $22,350." *Bangor Daily News*, January 12, 2012. http://bangordailynews.com/2012/01/12/health/lepage-plan-would-cut-mainecare-coverage-for-families-making-more-than-22350/.

Fellowes, Matthew, Virginia Gray, and David Lowery. 2006. "What's on the Table? The Content of State Policy Agendas." *Party Politics* 12 (January): 35–55.

Fox, Daniel M. 1999. "Strengthening State Government through Oversight." *Journal of Health Politics, Policy and Law* 24:1185–90.

Fox, Daniel M., and John K. Iglehart, eds. 1994. *Five States That Could Not Wait: Lessons for Health Reform from Florida, Hawaii, Minnesota, Oregon, and Vermont*. Cambridge, MA: Health Affairs and Milbank Memorial Fund.

Fox, Edward J. 1994. "States as Policy Laboratories: Health Care Policy Making, 1900–1994." Paper presented at Annual Meeting of American Political Science Association, New York, September.

Frendreis, John, and Richard Waterman. 1985. "PAC Contributions and Legislative Behavior: Senate Voting on Trucking Deregulation." *Social Science Quarterly* 66:401–12.

Fuchs, Victor R, and Ezekiel J. Emanuel. 2005. "Health Care Reform: Why? What? When?" *Health Affairs* 24 (6): 1399–1414.

Gabel, Jon R., Heidi Whitmore, and Jeremy Pickreign. 2008. "Market Watch: Report from Massachusetts: Employers Largely Support Health Care Reform, and Few Signs of Crowd-Out Appear." *Health Affairs* 27 (1): 13–23.

Gais, Thomas, and Jack Walker. 1991. "Pathways to Influence in American Politics." In *Mobilizing Interest Groups in America*, edited by Jack Walker Jr. Ann Arbor: University of Michigan Press.

General Accounting Office. 1997. *Managed Care: Explicit Gag Clauses Not Found in HMO Contracts, but Physician Concerns Remain.* Washington, DC: US Government Printing Office.

Gibson, Rosemary, and Janardan Prasad Singh. 2012. *The Battle over Health Care: What Obama's Reform Means for America's Future.* Lanham, MD: Rowman & Littlefield.

Glick, Henry R., and Scott P. Hays. 1991. "Innovation and Reinvention in State Policymaking: Theory and the Evolution of Living-Will Laws." *Journal of Politics* 53 (August): 835–50.

Godwin, Kenneth. 1988. *One Billion Dollars of Influence: The Direct Marketing of Politics.* New York: Chatham House.

Gold, Marsha R., Jessica Mittler, Anna Aizer, Barbara Lyons, and Cathy Schoen. 2001. "Health Insurance Expansion through States in a Pluralistic System." *Journal of Health Politics, Policy and Law* 26:581–614.

Gormley, William T., Jr. 1986. "Regulatory Issue Networks in a Federal System." *Polity* 18 (Summer): 595–620.

Gray, Virginia. 1973. "Innovation in the States: A Diffusion Study." *American Political Science Review* 67 (December): 1174–85.

Gray, Virginia, and David Lowery. 1988. "Interest Group Politics and Economic Growth in the US States." *American Political Science Review* 82:109–31.

———. 1995a. "The Demography of Interest Organization Communities: Institutions, Associations, and Membership Groups." *American Politics Quarterly* 23:3–32.

———. 1995b. "Interest Representation and Democratic Gridlock." *Legislative Studies Quarterly* 20 (4): 531–52.

———. 1996. *The Population Ecology of Interest Representation.* Ann Arbor: University of Michigan Press.

———. 1997. "Reconceptualizing PAC Formation: It's Not a Collective Action Problem, and It May Be an Arms Race." *American Politics Quarterly* 25:319–46.

———. 1998a. "The Density of State Interest Communities: Do Regional Variables Matter?" *Publius* 28:61–79.

———. 1998b. "State Lobbying Regulations and Their Enforcement: Implications for the Diversity of State Interest Communities." *State and Local Government Review* 30 (2): 78–91.

———. 2001. "The Institutionalization of State Communities of Organized Interests." *Political Research Quarterly* 54 (2): 265–84.

Gray, Virginia, David Lowery, Matthew Fellowes, and Jennifer Anderson. 2005a. "Legislative Agendas and Interest Advocacy: Understanding the Demand Side of Lobbying." *American Politics Research* 33 (3): 404–34.

Gray, Virginia, David Lowery, and Erik Godwin. 2007a. "The Political Management of Managed Care: Explaining Variations in State Health Maintenance Organizations Regulations." *Journal of Health Politics, Policy and Law* 32 (June): 457–95.

———. 2007b. "Public Preferences and Organized Interests in Health Policy: State Pharmacy Assistance Programs as Innovations." *Journal of Health Politics, Policy and Law* 32 (February): 82–113.

Gray, Virginia, David Lowery, James Monogan, and Erik Godwin. 2011. "Incrementing toward Nowhere: Universal Health Care Coverage in the States," *Publius* 40 (1).

Gray, Virginia, David Lowery, Jennifer Wolak, Erik Godwin, and Whitt Kilburn. 2005b. "Reconsidering the Countermobilization Hypothesis: Health Policy Lobbying in the American States." *Political Behavior* 27:99–132.

Greenblatt, Alan. 2011. "Right-Minded." *Governing*, December, 32–36.

Grenzke, Janet. 1989. "PACs and the Congressional Supermarket: The Currency Is Complex." *American Journal of Political Science* 33:1–24.

Grier, Kevin B., Michael C. Munger, and Brian E. Roberts. 1994. "The Determinants of Industry Political Activity, 1978–1986." *American Political Science Review* 88:911–26.

Grogan, Colleen M. 1993. "Federalism and Health Care Reform." *American Behavioral Scientist* 36:741–59.

———. 1994. "Political-Economic Factors Influencing State Medicaid Policy." *Political Research Quarterly* 47:589–622.

Grossback, Lawrence J., Sean Nicholson-Crotty, and David A. M. Peterson. 2004. "Ideology and Learning in Policy Diffusion." *American Politics Research* 32 (September): 521–45.

Grossman, Matt. 2012. *The Not-So-Special Interests: Interest Groups, Public Representation, and American Governance.* Stanford, CA: Stanford University Press.

Group Health. 1991. *An Enduring Mission: The Story of Group Health.* Saint Paul: Group Health, Inc.

Haberkorn, Jennifer. 2010. "States Wary of High-Risk Pools." *Politico*, April, 27. www.politico.com/news/stories/0410/36374.html.

Hacker, Jacob S. 2010. "The Road to Somewhere: Why Health Reform Happened." *Perspectives on Politics* 8 (September): 861–76.

———. 2011. "Why Reform Happened." *Journal of Health Politics, Policy and Law* 36 (June): 437–41.

Hackey, Robert B., and David A. Rochefort, eds. 2001. *The New Politics of State Health Policy.* Lawrence: University Press of Kansas.

Haeder, Simon F. 2012. "Beyond Path Dependence: Explaining Healthcare Reform and Its Consequences." *Policy Studies Journal* 40 (S1): 65–86.

Hall, Mark A. 2005. "The Death of Managed Care: A Regulatory Autopsy." *Journal of Health Politics, Policy and Law* 30:427–52.

Hall, Mark A., and G. Agrawal. 2003. "The Impact of State-Managed Care Liability Statutes." *Health Affairs* 22 (5): 138–45.

Hall, Richard J., and Robert P. Van Houweling. 2006. "Campaign Contributions and Lobbying on the Medicare Modernization Act of 2003." Paper prepared for delivery at Annual Meeting of American Political Science Association, Philadelphia, August 30–September 3.

Halpin, Darren, and Grant Jordan. 2009. "Interpreting Environments: Interest Group Response to Population Ecology Pressures." *British Journal of Political Science* 39:243–65.

Halpin, Helen A., and Peter Harbage. 2010. "The Origins and Demise of the Public Option." *Health Affairs* 29 (June): 1117–24.

Hannan, Michael T., and Glenn R. Carroll. 1992. *Dynamics of Organizational Populations.* New York: Oxford University Press.

Hansen, John Mark. 1985. "The Political Economy of Group Membership." *American Political Science Review* 79 (1): 79–96.

Harkness, Peter A. 2012. "Judgment Time on Health Care." *Governing*, May, 16–17.

Havighurst, Clark C. 2002. "How the Health Care Revolution Fell Short." *Law & Contemporary Problems* 65 (4): 55–101.

Hays, Scott P. 1996. "Influences on Reinvention during the Diffusion of Innovations." *Political Research Quarterly* 49 (3): 631–50.

Heaney, Michael T. 2006. "Brokering Health Policy: Coalitions, Parties, and Interest Group Influence." *Journal of Health Politics, Policy and Law* 31 (October): 887–944.

Heinz, John P., Edward O. Laumann, Robert L. Nelson, and Robert Salisbury. 1993. *The Hollow Core.* Cambridge, MA: Harvard University Press.

Henry J. Kaiser Family Foundation. 2012. *Health Care Costs: A Primer.* www .kff.org/insurance/upload/7670-03.pdf.

Hernandez, Raymond, and Robert Pear. 2004. "State Officials Are Cautious on Medicare Drug Benefit." *New York Times*, January 4. www.nytimes .com/2004/01/04/us/state-officials-are-cautious-on-medicare-drug-benefit .html.

Holahan, John, and Irene Headen. 2010. "Medicaid Coverage and Spending in Health Reform: National and State-by-State Results for Adults at or Below 133% FPL." Kaiser Commission on Medicaid and the Uninsured. www.kff.org/healthreform/upload/medicaid-coverage-and-spending-in- health-reform-national-and-state-by-state-results-for-adults-at-or-below- 133-fpl.pdf.

Holahan, John, and Mary Beth Pohl. 2003. "Leaders and Laggards in State Coverage Expansions." In *Federalism and Health Policy*, edited by John Holahan, Alan Weil, and Joshua M. Wiener. Washington, DC: Urban Institute Press.

Hovey, Kendra A., and Harold A. Hovey. 2004. *CQ's State Fact Finder 2004.* Washington, DC: CQ Press.

Isikoff, Michael. 2011. "White House Used Mitt Romney Health Care Law as Blueprint for Federal Law." MSNBC, October 11. www.msnbc.msn.com/ id/44854320/nx/politics-decision_2012/t/white-house-used-mitt-romney -health-care-law-blueprint-federal-law/?nw=politics-decision_2012#.

Jacobs, Lawrence R. 2010. "What Health Reform Teaches Us about American Politics." *PS* 43 (October): 619–23.

———. 2011. "America's Critical Juncture: The Affordable Care Act and Its Reverberations." *Journal of Health Politics, Policy and Law* 36 (June): 625–31.

Jacobs, Lawrence R., and Robert Y. Shapiro. 1999. "The American Public's Pragmatic Liberalism Meets Its Philosophical Conservatism." *Journal of Health Politics, Policy and Law* 24 (5): 1021–31.

Jacobs, Lawrence R., and Theda Skocpol. 2010. *Health Care Reform and American Politics: What Everyone Needs to Know.* New York: Oxford University Press.

Jamieson, Kathleen Hall. 1994. *The Role of Advertising in the Health Care Debate*, parts 1–3. Philadelphia: University of Pennsylvania.

Johnson, Haynes, and David S. Broder. 1996. *The System: The American Way of Politics at the Breaking Point.* Boston: Little, Brown.

Jones, Bryan D., and Frank Baumgartner. 2005. *The Politics of Attention: How Governments Prioritize Problems.* Chicago: University of Chicago Press.

Jones, Bryan D., Tracy Sulkin, and Heather A. Larsen. 2003. "Policy Punctuations in American Political Institutions." *American Political Science Review* 97:151–69.

Jones, David K., Katharine W. V. Bradley, and Jonathan Oberlander. 2012. "Pascal's Wager: Health Insurance Exchanges and the Republican Dilemma." Paper presented at Annual Meeting of Midwest Political Science Association, Chicago, April.

Jost, Timothy S. 2010. "State Lawsuits Won't Succeed in Overturning the Individual Mandate." *Health Affairs* 29 (June): 1225–28.

Kaiser State Health Facts. 2012a. "Insurer Rebates under the Medical Loss Ratio: 2012 Estimates." www.kff.org/healthreform/8305.cfm.

———. 2012b. "State Decisions for Creating Health Insurance Exchanges in 2014 as of December 14, 2012." www.statehealthfacts.org/comparemaptable .jsp?ind=962&cat=17.

———. 2012c. "Total Health Insurance Exchange Grants, 2012." www .statehealthfacts.org/comparetable.jsp?ind=964&cat=17.

Karch, Andrew. 2007. *Democratic Laboratories: Policy Diffusion among the American States.* Ann Arbor: University of Michigan Press.

Key, V. O. 1949. *Southern Politics.* New York: Alfred A. Knopf.

Kim, Ae-sook, and Edward Jennings. 2012. "The Evolution of an Innovation: Variations in Medicaid Managed Care Program Extensiveness." *Journal of Health Politics, Policy and Law* 37 (October): 815–49.

King, Martha. 2010. "Forecast for States on Medicaid Expension." *State Legislatures* 27 (October–November): 27.

Kingdon, John W. 2011. *Agendas, Alternatives, and Public Policies, Updated 2nd ed.* Boston: Longman.

Kinney, Eleanor DeArman. 2002. *Protecting American Health Care Consumers.* Durham, NC: Duke University Press.

Kliff, Sarah. 2011. "Some States Seek Flexibility to Push Health-Care Overhaul Further." *Washington Post*, October 17.

Konisky, David, and Lilliard E. Richardson Jr. 2012. "Penalizing the Party: Health Care Reform Issue Voting in the 2010 Election." *American Politics Research*, Doi:10.1177/1532673X11434141/apr.sagepub.com.

Kousser, Thad. 2002. "The Politics of Discretionary Medicaid Spending, 1980–1993." *Journal of Health Politics, Policy and Law* 27:639–71.

Kronebusch, Karl, Mark Schlesinger, and Tracey Thomas. 2009. "Managed Care Regulation in the States: The Impact on Physicians' Practices and Clinical Autonomy." *Journal of Health, Politics, Policy and Law* 34 (April): 219–59.

Lamothe, Scott. 2005. "State Policy Adoption and Content: A Study of Drug Testing in the Workplace Legislation." *State and Local Government Review* 37:25–39.

Leichter, Howard M., ed. 1997a. *Health Policy Reform in America: Innovations from the States, 2nd Edition.* Armonk, NY: M. E. Sharpe.

———. 1997b. "The Little State That Could—Couldn't: Vermont Stumbles on the Road to Reform." In *Health Policy Reform in America: Innovations from the States, 2nd Edition*, edited by Howard M. Leichter. Armonk, NY: M. E. Sharpe.

———. 2004. "Obstacles to Dependent Health Care Access in Oregon: Health Insurance or Health Care?" *Journal of Health Politics, Policy and Law* 29 (April): 237–68.

Lester, James P., James Franke, Ann O'M. Bowman, and Kenneth Kramer. 1983. "Hazardous Waste Politics and Public Policy: A Comparative State Analysis." *Western Political Science Quarterly* 36:257–85.

Long, Sharon K., and Karen Stockley. 2010. "Sustaining Health Reform in a Recession: An Update on Massachusetts as of Fall 2009." *Health Affairs* 29 (June): 1234–41.

Lowery, David, and Holly Brasher. 2004. *Organized Interests and American Government.* Boston: McGraw-Hill.

Lowery, David, and Virginia Gray. 1994. "Do Lobbying Regulations Influence Lobbying Registrations?" *Social Science Quarterly* 75 (2): 382–84.

———. 1997. "How Some Rules Just Don't Matter: The Regulation of Lobbyists." *Public Choice* 91:139–47.

———. 2004a. "Bias in the Heavenly Chorus: Interests in Society and Before Government." *Journal of Theoretical Politics* 16 (1): 5–30.

———. 2004b. "A Neopluralist Perspective on Research on Organized Interests." *Political Research Quarterly* 57 (1): 163–75.

———. 2007. "Understanding Interest System Diversity: Health Interest Communities in the American States." *Business and Politics* 9, article 2.

Lowery, David, Virginia Gray, and Frank R. Baumgartner. 2011. "Policy Attention in State and Nation: Is Anyone Listening to the Laboratories of Democracy?" *Publius: The Journal of Federalism* 41 (Spring): 1–25.

Lowery, David, Virginia Gray, Jennifer Benz, Mary Deason, Justin Kirkland, and Jennifer Sykes. 2009. "Understanding the Relationship between Health PACs and Health Lobbying in the American States." *Publius* 39 (Winter): 70–94.

Lowery, David, Virginia Gray, and Matthew Fellowes. 2005. "Sisyphus Meets the Borg: Understanding the Diversity of Interest Communities." *Journal of Theoretical Politics* 17 (1): 41–74.

Lowery, David, Virginia Gray, Matthew Fellowes, and Jennifer Anderson. 2004. "Living in the Moment: Lags, Leads, and the Link between Legislative Agendas and Interest Advocacy." *Social Science Quarterly* 85 (2): 463–77.

Mahoney, Christine. 2003. "Following the Pack: Bandwagons in State Policy Innovation Diffusion." Unpublished manuscript, Department of Political Science, Pennsylvania State University.

Managed Care On-Line. 2009. "Managed Care National Statistics." www .mcareol.com/factshts/factnati.htm.

Mathews, Anna Wilde, and Avery Johnson. 2010. "Insurer Fights Maine Regulator on Premiums." *Wall Street Journal*, April 2. http://online.wsj .com/article/SB10001424052748704059004575127533188447508. html.

Mayes, Rick. 2004. *Universal Coverage: The Elusive Quest for National Health Insurance.* Ann Arbor: University of Michigan Press.

McDonough, John E. 1992. "States First: The Other Path to National Health Reform." *American Prospect* 9:61–66.

———. 2011. *Inside National Health Reform.* Berkeley: University of California Press/Milbank Memorial Fund.

McFarland, Andrew S. 2004. *Neopluralism.* Lawrence: University of Kansas Press.

McVoy, Edgar C. 1940. "Patterns of Diffusion in the United States." *American Sociological Review* 5 (April): 219–27.

Meier, Kenneth, and Gary W. Copeland. 1984. "Pass the Biscuits Pappy: Congressional Decision-Making and Federal Grants." *American Politics Quarterly* 12 (1): 3–21.

Meier, Kenneth J., and E. Thomas Garman. 1995. *Regulation and Consumer Protection, 2nd Ed.* Houston: Dame Publications.

Messer, Anne, Joost Berkhout, and David Lowery. 2011. "The Density of the EU Interest System: A Test of the ESA Model." *British Journal of Political Science* 41 (1): 161–90.

Milbank Memorial Fund and Reforming States Group. 1999. *Tracking State*

Oversight of Managed Care. www.milbank.org/stateoversight/990918soihs .html.

Miller, Edward A. 2004. "Advancing Comparative State Policy Research: Toward Conceptual Interaction and Methodological Expansion." *State and Local Government Review* 36 (1): 35–58.

———. 2005. "State Health Policy Making Determinants, Theory, and Methods: A Synthesis." *Social Science & Medicine* 61 (12): 2639–57.

———. 2006. "Explaining Incremental and Non-Incremental Change: Medicaid Nursing Facility Reimbursement Policy, 1980–98." *State Politics and Policy Quarterly* 6 (2): 117–50.

Miller, Michael, and Brian Rosman. 2004. "Dirigo Health: What Does Maine's New Health Care Law Mean for Other States?" www.communitycatalyst .org/doc_store/publications/what_does_maines_new_health_care_law_ mean_for_other_states_feb04.pdf.

Miller, Tracy E. 1997. "Managed Care Regulation: In the Laboratory of the States." *Journal of the American Medical Association* 278 (13): 1102–9.

Mintrom, Michael. 1997. "Policy Entrepreneurs and the Diffusion of Innovation." *American Journal of Political Science* 41:738–70.

Mistler, Steve. 2010. "LePage Team Says Dirigo Will Be Replaced When It's 'Diri-Gone.'" *Sun Journal* (Lewiston, ME), November 11. www.sunjournal .com/state/story/940697.

Moe, Terry M. 1980. *The Organization of Interests.* Chicago: University of Chicago Press.

Mohr, Lawrence B. 1969. "Determinants of Innovation in Organizations." *American Political Science Review* 63:111–26.

Monson, State Senator Angela. 2001. "Testimony on Behalf of the National Conference of State Legislatures before the Subcommittee on Health, Committee on Energy and Commerce, US House of Representatives, on March 15." www.ncsl.org/programs/press/2001/monson-pbor.htm.

Morgan, Kimberly J., and Andrea Louise Campbell. 2011a. "Delegated Governance in the Affordable Care Act." *Journal of Health Politics, Policy and Law* 36 (June): 387–91.

———. 2011b. *The Delegated Welfare State: Medicare, Markets, and the Governance of Social Policy.* New York: Oxford University Press.

Mulholland, Jessica. 2010. "California: A National Model for Health Benefit Exchanges?" *Governing,* November. www.governing.com/topics/health-human-services/California-national-model-health-benefit-exchanges .html.

NBC Nightly News. 2009. "What's a Health Care Co-op?" August.

NCSL (National Conference of State Legislatures). 2004. "State Pharmaceutical Assistance Programs, 2004 Edition." www.ncsl.org/programs/health/drugaid.htm.

———. 2005. "Universal Health Care Legislation: History and Archive, 1975 to 2004." www.ncsl.org/default.aspx?tabid=14068.

———. 2007. "Health Reform Bills, 2007." www.ncsl.org/Default.aspx?TabId=14356

———. 2009. "State Pharmaceutical Assistance Programs, 2009 Edition." www.ncsl.org/programs/health/drugaid.htm.

———. 2010a. "State Legislation and Actions Challenging Certain Health Reforms, 2010." www.ncsl.org/?tabid=18906.

———. 2010b. "State Legislation Challenging Certain Health Reforms, 2010." www.ncsl.org/default.aspx?tabid=18906.

———. 2010c. "State Pharmaceutical Assistance Programs." www.ncsl.org/default.aspx?tabid=14334.

———. 2011. "State Legislation and Actions Challenging Certain Health Reforms, 2011." www.ncsl.org/?tabid=18906.

———. 2012. "State Legislation and Actions Challenging Certain Health Reforms, 2011–2012." www.ncsl.org/issues-research/health/state-laws-and-actions-challenging-aca.aspx.

Neubauer, Deane. 1997. "Hawaii: The Health State Revisited." In *Health Policy Reform in America: Innovations from the States, 2nd Edition*, edited by Howard M. Leichter. Armonk, NY: M. E. Sharpe.

Nice, David C. 1994. *Policy Innovation in State Government*. Ames: Iowa State University Press.

Nicholson-Crotty, Sean. 2009. "The Politics of Diffusion: Public Policy in the American States." *Journal of Politics* 71 (January): 192–205.

Noble, A. A., and T. A. Brennan. 1999. "The Stages of Managed Care Regulation: Developing Better Rules." *Journal of Health Politics, Policy and Law* 24:1275–1306.

Nownes, Anthony. 2000. "The Structure of Interest Communities: A Comparative State Analysis." *American Politics Quarterly* 28 (July): 309–27.

———. 2004. "The Population Ecology of Interest Group Formation: Mobilizing for Gay and Lesbian Rights in the United States, 1950–1998." *British Journal of Political Science* 28:49–76.

Nownes, Anthony, and Paul Freeman. 1998. "Interest Group Activity in the States." *Journal of Politics* 60 (February): 86–112.

Nownes, Anthony, and Daniel Lapinski. 2005. "The Population Ecology of

Interest Group Death: Gay and Lesbian Rights Interest Groups in the United States, 1948–1998." *British Journal of Political Science* 35 (April): 303–19.

Oberlander, Jonathan. 2007. "Through the Looking Glass: The Politics of the Medicare Prescription Drug, Improvement, and Modernization Act." *Journal of Health Politics, Policy and Law* 32 (April): 187–219.

———. 2010. "Long Time Coming: Why Health Reform Finally Passed." *Health Affairs* 29 (June): 1112–16.

Oliver, Thomas R. 2004. "Policy Entrepreneurship in the Social Transformation of American Medicine: The Rise of Managed Care and Managed Competition." *Journal of Health Politics, Policy and Law* 29 (4–5): 701–34.

Oliver, Thomas R., Philip R. Lee, and Helene L. Lipton. 2004. "A Political History of Medicare and Prescription Drug Coverage." *Milbank Quarterly* 82 (2): 283–354.

Oliver, Thomas R., and Pamela Paul-Shaheen. 1997. "Translating Ideas into Actions: Entrepreneurial Leadership in State Health Care Reforms." *Journal of Health Politics, Policy and Law* 22 (3): 721–89.

Olson, Mancur, Jr. 1965. *The Logic of Collective Action.* Cambridge, MA: Harvard University Press.

———. 1982. *The Rise and Decline of Nations: Economic Growth, Stagflation, and Social Rigidities.* New Haven, CT: Yale University Press.

Pacheco, Julianna. 2012. "The Social Contagion Model: Exploring the Role of Public Opinion on the Diffusion of Antismoking Legislation across the American States." *Journal of Politics* 74 (1): 187–202.

Patel, Kavita, and John McDonough. 2010. "From Massachusetts to 1600 Pennsylvania Avenue: Aboard the Health Reform Express." *Health Affairs* 29 (June): 1106–11.

Paul-Shaheen, Pamela A. 1998. "The States and Health Care Reform: The Road Traveled and Lessons Learned from Seven That Took the Lead." *Journal of Health Politics, Policy and Law* 23 (April): 319–61.

Pear, Robert. 2010. "Health Care Overhaul Depends on States' Insurance Exchanges." *New York Times*, October 23.

———. 2011. "Health Care Law Will Let States Tailor Benefits." *New York Times*, December 16. www.nytimes.com/2011/12/17/health/policy/health-care-law-to-allow-states-to-pick-benefits.html?sq=Robert%20Pear&st=cse=scp=10&pagewanted=print.

Peltzman, Sam. 1976. "Towards a More General Theory of Regulation." *Journal of Law and Economics* 19:211–40.

Peterson, Mark A. 1995. "The Health Care Debate: All Heat and No Light." *Journal of Health Politics, Policy and Law* 20 (Summer): 225–230.

———. 2011. "It Was a Different Time: Obama and the Unique Opportunity for Health Care Reform." *Journal of Health Politics, Policy and Law* 36 (June): 429–36.

Pracht, Etieene E. 2007. "State Medicaid Managed Care Enrollment: Understanding the Political Calculus That Drives Medicaid Managed Care Reforms." *Journal of Health Politics, Policy and Law* 32 (August): 685–731.

Pracht, Etieene E., and William J. Moore. 2003. "Interest Groups and State Medicaid Drug Programs." *Journal of Health Politics, Policy and Law* 28 (1): 9–30.

Quadagno, Jill. 2005. *One Nation Uninsured.* New York: Oxford University Press.

———. 2011. "Interest-Group Influence on the Patient Protection and Affordability Act of 2010: Winners and Losers in the Health Care Reform Debate." *Journal of Health Politics, Policy and Law* 36 (June): 449–53.

Quinn, Dennis, and Robert Shapiro. 1991. "Business Political Power: The Case of Taxation." *American Political Science Review* 85 (September): 852–74.

Reforming States Group. 2003. "State Initiatives on Prescription Drugs: Creating a More Functional Market." *Health Affairs* 22 (4): 128–36.

Robinson, James C. 2001. "The End of Managed Care." *Journal of the American Medical Association* 285:2622–28.

———. 2003. "The Politics of Managed Competition: Public Abuse of the Private Interest." *Journal of Health Politics, Policy and Law* 28 (April–June): 341–53.

Rogers, Everett M. 2003. *Diffusion of Innovations, 5th Edition.* New York: Free Press.

Rosenstone, Steven J., and John Mark Hansen. 1993. *Mobilization, Participation, and Democracy in America.* New York: Macmillan.

Rosenthal, Meredith. 2004. "Market Watch: Doughnut-Hole Economics." *Health Affairs* 23 (6): 129–35.

Ross, E. Clarke. 1999. "Regulating Managed Care: Interest Group Competition for Control and Behavioral Health Care." *Journal of Health Politics, Policy and Law* 24 (3): 599–614.

Sack, Kevin. 2007. "States' Widening of Health Care Hits Roadblocks." *New York Times*, December 25. Available at www.nytimes.com.

———. 2009a. "Health Co-Op Offers Model for Overhaul." *New York Times*, July 7. Available at www.nytimes.com.

———. 2009b. "Massachusetts Faces Costs of Big Health Care Plan." *New York Times*, March 16. Available at www.nytimes.com.

Salisbury, Robert H. 1969. "An Exchange Theory of Interest Groups." *Midwest Journal of Political Science* 13 (February): 1–32.

Sapat, Alka. 2004. "Devolution and Innovation: The Adoption of State Environmental Policy Innovations by Administrative Agencies." *Public Administration Review* 64 (March–April): 141–51.

Satterthwaite, Shad. 2002. "Innovation and Diffusion of Managed Care in Medicaid Programs." *State and Local Government Review* 34:116–26.

Schattschneider, E. E. 1960. *The Semisovereign People*. New York: Holt, Rinehart, and Winston.

Schlozman, Kay Lehman, and John T. Tierney. 1986. *Organized Interests and American Democracy*. New York: Harper & Row.

Schlozman, Kay Lehman, Sidney Verba, and Henry E. Brady. 2012. *The Unheavenly Chorus: Unequal Political Voice and the Broken Promise of American Democracy*. Princeton, NJ: Princeton University Press.

Scott, Dylan. 2012. "Supreme Court Ruling: Uncertain Future for Medicaid Expansion." Governing.com blog, June 28. www.governing.com/blogs/view/gov-supreme-court-ruling-uncertain-future-for-aca-medicaid-expansion.html.

Sebok, Anthony J. 2004. "The Supreme Court Rejects State Law Suits Challenging Health Coverage: Why the Ruling May Spawn an Election Issue." www.findlaw.com/sebok/20040628.html.

Serafini, Marilyn Weber. 2003. "Health Care—No Cure—All Key Provisions of the Medicare Bill." *National Journal*, November 22. Available at www.NationalJournal.com.

———. 2009a. "Harry and Louise: The Sequel." *National Journal*, July 18, 28.

———. 2009b. "The Lessons of Massachusetts." *National Journal*, July 18, 22–26.

Shapiro, Ilya. 2010. "State Suits against Health Reform Are Well Grounded in Law—and Pose Serious Challenges." *Health Affairs* 29 (June): 1229–33.

Shipan, Charles R., and Craig Volden. 2006. "Bottom-Up Federalism: The Diffusion of Antismoking Policies from US Cities to States." *American Journal of Political Science* 50 (October): 825–43.

Sigelman, Lee, David Lowery, and Roland Smith. 1983. "The Tax Revolt: A Comparative State Analysis." *Western Political Quarterly* 6 (March): 30–51.

Skocpol, Theda. 1996. *Boomerang: Clinton's Health Security Effort and the Turn against Government in US. Politics*. New York: W. W. Norton.

———. 2010. "The Political Challenges That May Undermine Health Reform." *Health Affairs* 29 (7): 1288–92.

Smith, Mark A. 2000. *American Business and Political Power.* Chicago: University of Chicago.

Sorian, Richard, and Judith Feder. 1999. "Why We Need a Patients' Bill of Rights." *Journal of Health Politics, Policy and Law* 24 (5): 1137–44.

Spatz, Ian D. 2010. "Health Reform Accelerates Changes in the Pharmaceutical Industry." *Health Affairs* 29 (July): 1331–36. http://content.healthaffairs.org/cgi/reprint/29/7/1331.

"Special Issue: Insurance Coverage and the States." 2004. *Journal of Health Politics, Policy and Law* 29.

Starr, Paul. 1982. *The Social Transformation of American Medicine: The Rise of a Sovereign Profession and the Making of a Vast New Industry.* New York: Basic Books.

———. 2011. *Remedy and Reaction: The Peculiar American Struggle over Health Care Reform.* New Haven, CT: Yale University Press.

Steinmo, Sven, and Jon Watts. 1995. "It's the Institutions, Stupid! Why Comprehensive National Health Insurance Always Fails in America." *Journal of Health Politics, Policy, and Law* 20:329–71.

Stigler, George. 1971. "The Theory of Economic Regulation." *Bell Journal of Economics and Management Science* 2:3–21.

Stolberg, Sheryl Gay, and Kevin Sack. 2011. "Obama Backs Easing State Health Law Mandates." *New York Times*, February 28. www.nytimes.com/2011/03/01/us/politics/01health.html?_r=1&sq=Stolberg%20and%20Sack%20March%201%202011&st=cse&scp=1&pagewanted=print.

Stone, Deborah. 1999. "Managed Care and the Second Great Transformation." *Journal of Health Politics, Policy and Law* 24 (5): 1213–18.

Stream, Christopher. 1999. "Health Reform in the States: A Model of State Small Group Health Insurance Market Reforms." *Political Research Quarterly* 52 (3): 499–525.

Stych, Ed. 1992. "AMA Seeks a Truce with Archrival HMOs." *Seattle Community Times,* June 11, 1992. http://community.seattletimes.nwsource.com/archive/?date=19920611&slug=1496623.

Teske, Paul. 2004. *Regulation in the States.* Washington, DC: Brookings Institution Press.

Thompson, Frank J., and Courtney Burke. 2007. "Executive Federalism and Medicaid Demonstration Waivers: Implications for Policy and Democratic Process." *Journal of Health Politics, Policy and Law* 32 (December): 971–1004.

Titlow, Karen, and Ezekiel Emanuel. 1999. "Employer Decisions and the Seeds of Backlash." *Journal of Health Politics, Policy and Law* 24 (5): 941–47.

Trail, Thomas, Kimberley Fox, Joel Cantor, Mina Silberberg, and Stephen Crystal. 2004. *State Pharmacy Assistance Programs: A Chartbook*. New Brunswick, NJ: Rutgers Center for State Health Policy. www.common wealthfund.org/~/media/Files/Publications/Chartbook/2004/Aug/ State%20Pharmacy%20Assistance%20Programs%20%20A%20 Chartbook/758_Trail_state_pharmacy_assist_progs_chartb2%20pdf.pdf.

Tripathi, Micky, Stephen Ansolabehere, and James Snyder. 2002. "Are PAC Contributions and Lobbying Linked? New Evidence from the 1995 Lobby Disclosure Act." *Business and Politics* 4:131–55.

Truman, David. 1951. *The Governmental Process*. New York: Alfred A. Knopf.

Van Denburg, Hart. 2010. "Tim Pawlenty Orders Minnesota Not to Access Federal Health Care Reform Money." August 31. http://blogs.citypages .com/blotter/2010/08/tim_pawlenty_de_2.php?print=true.

Vermont Campaign for Health Care Security Education Fund. 2009. "History of Vermont Medicaid / Dr. Dynasaur/Pharmacy Eligibility Expansions since 1986." www.catamounthealth.org/catamount-health-expansion.htm.

Volden, Craig. 2006. "States as Policy Laboratories: Emulating Success in the Children's Health Insurance Program." *American Journal of Political Science* 50:294–312.

Walker, Jack L. 1969. "The Diffusion of Innovations among the American States." *American Political Science Review* 13:880–99.

———. 1991. *Mobilizing Interest Groups in America: Patrons, Professionals, and Social Movements*. Ann Arbor: University of Michigan Press.

Weil, Alan, and Raymond Scheppach. 2010. "New Roles for States in Health Reform Implementation." *Health Affairs* 29 (June): 1178–82.

Weissert, Carol S., and Daniel Scheller. 2008. "Learning from the States? Federalism and National Health Policy." *Public Administration Review* December Special Issue: S162-S174.

Weissert, Carol S., and William G. Weissert. 1996. *Governing Health: The Politics of Health Policy*. Baltimore: Johns Hopkins University Press.

———. 2002. *Governing Health: The Politics of Health Policy, 2nd Edition*. Baltimore: Johns Hopkins University Press.

———. 2006. *Governing Health: The Politics of Health Policy, 3rd Edition*. Baltimore: Johns Hopkins University Press.

Weissert, William G., and Edward Alan Miller. 2005. "Punishing the Pioneers: The Medicare Modernization Act and State Pharmacy Assistance Programs." *Publius: The Journal of Federalism* 35 (Winter): 115–41.

Welch, Susan, and Kay Thompson. 1980. "The Impact of Federal Incentives on State Policy Innovation." *American Journal of Political Science* 24 (November): 715–29.

West, Darrell M., Diane Heith, and Chris Goodwin. 1996. "Harry and Louise Go to Washington: Political Advertising and Health Care Reform." *Journal of Health Politics, Policy, and Law* 21:35–68.

West, Darrell M., and Burdett A. Loomis. 1999. *The Sound of Money.* New York: W. W. Norton.

Whitaker, Eric A., Mitchel N. Herian, Christopher W. Larimer, and Michael Lang. 2012. "The Determinants of Policy Introduction and Bill Adoption: Examining Minimum Wage Increases in the American States, 1997–2006." *Policy Studies Journal* 40 (4): 626–49.

Wilhite, Allen, and John Theilmann. 1987. "Labor PAC Contributions and Labor Legislation: A Simultaneous Logit Approach." *Public Choice* 53:277–84.

Wolfe, Warren. 2011. "95,000 Poor Minnesotans Will Get Medicaid Today." *Minneapolis Star Tribune*, January 5. Available at www.StarTribune.com.

Wright, Jack. 1985. "PACs, Contributions, and Roll Calls: An Organizational Perspective." *American Political Science Review* 79:400–414.

———. 2004. "Campaign Contributions and Congressional Voting on Tobacco Policy, 1980–2000." *Business and Politics* 6:1–26.

Yackee, Susan Webb. 2009. "Private Conflict and Policy Passage: Interest Group Conflict and State Medical Malpractice Reform." *Policy Studies Journal* 37 (May): 213–31.

INDEX